Low Back Pain and Sciatica

AF382693

Luigi Tesio

Low Back Pain and Sciatica

A New Pathogenetic Model and Treatment Principles

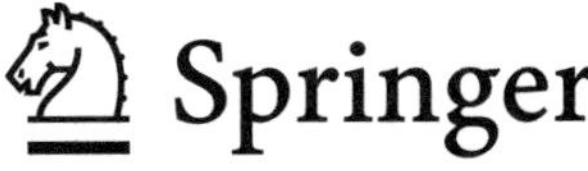 Springer

Luigi Tesio
Dept. of Neurorehabilitation Sciences
Istituto Auxologico Italiano, IRCCS
University of Milan
Milano, Italy

ISBN 978-3-031-78536-8   ISBN 978-3-031-78534-4   (eBook)
https://doi.org/10.1007/978-3-031-78534-4

The original submitted manuscript has been translated into English. The translation was done using artificial intelligence. A subsequent revision was performed by the author(s) to further refine the work and to ensure that the translation is appropriate concerning content and scientific correctness. It may, however, read stylistically different from a conventional translation.

Translation from the Italian language edition: "Il dolore lombosciatico. Un nuovo modello patogenetico e principi di trattamento" by Luigi Tesio, © Il Pensiero Scientifico Editore 2024. Published by Il Pensiero Scientifico Editore. All Rights Reserved.

© The Editor(s) (if applicable) and The Author(s), under exclusive license to Springer Nature Switzerland AG 2025
This work is subject to copyright. All rights are solely and exclusively licensed by the Publisher, whether the whole or part of the material is concerned, specifically the rights of reprinting, reuse of illustrations, recitation, broadcasting, reproduction on microfilms or in any other physical way, and transmission or information storage and retrieval, electronic adaptation, computer software, or by similar or dissimilar methodology now known or hereafter developed.
The use of general descriptive names, registered names, trademarks, service marks, etc. in this publication does not imply, even in the absence of a specific statement, that such names are exempt from the relevant protective laws and regulations and therefore free for general use.
The publisher, the authors and the editors are safe to assume that the advice and information in this book are believed to be true and accurate at the date of publication. Neither the publisher nor the authors or the editors give a warranty, expressed or implied, with respect to the material contained herein or for any errors or omissions that may have been made. The publisher remains neutral with regard to jurisdictional claims in published maps and institutional affiliations.

This Springer imprint is published by the registered company Springer Nature Switzerland AG
The registered company address is: Gewerbestrasse 11, 6330 Cham, Switzerland

If disposing of this product, please recycle the paper.

Foreword

It is with great surprise and a mix of pride and fear that I received the invitation from Professor Luigi Tesio to write a presentation for his book. The explanation for this set of feelings arises primarily from my consideration, undoubtedly shared by the entire scientific community, of Professor Tesio as an eminent Doctor (with a capital D), clinician, researcher and, therefore overall, a true scientist, with whom I share field experience (shared patients and problems) but also a long-standing connection that sees our doctoral dissertations written in the same area of interest, neurophysiology.

No less engaging was realizing the book's theme, namely lumbosciatica: a topic of extreme difficulty and very high frequency in everyday practice for physiatrists, neurosurgeons, neurologists, orthopedists, and colleagues in general medicine. In this regard, see the numbers of outpatient visits for this aptly defined "silent epidemic." I confess that I feared I might be in diametrically opposite positions (neurosurgeon-physiatrist war?). Instead, it was a pleasant surprise to see that the positions on diagnosis, clinical, and treatment considerations coincided on most points.

The diagnosis and understanding of pain mechanisms, an experience that is subjective "par excellence," can represent a genuine clinical and radiological dilemma, especially in an ageing population. Luigi Tesio's book seeks an objective and scientific answer to all this and a theory developed by the author himself, which is innovative and extremely interesting.

I am sure that this book represents an essential tool and is of rare importance for all doctors, from the youngest to the most experienced. I therefore hope that it represents a milestone present in all medical premises.

Professor of Neurosurgery
University of Milan
Milan, Italy

Unit of Neurosurgery
IRCCS Ca' Granda
Ospedale Maggiore Policlinico Foundation
Milan, Italy

Marco Locatelli

Introduction

There are very few adults who, during their lifetime, have not suffered from pain in the lumbar area or the classic "back pain" or pain along a lower limb. Almost always, these people will have received a diagnosis of "lumbago" or, in the second case, "sciatica" or even "limbo-sciatica". For brevity from here on, I will sometimes use the term lumbago (the familiar back pain or low-back pain, sometimes backache) also to include sciatica, lumbago-sciatica, and diffuse pains to the groin or the anterior face of the thigh, more appropriately defined as "cruralgia" (from the Latin "crus", leg: but indicating the root of the limb, the thigh): I will leave it to the context to specify the meaning.

I anticipate that I will use the noun "patient" to generally indicate the suffering person: in my experience, there is no significant gender difference between the age of onset, prevalence, type, and severity of this pathology. The duplication of gender (he/she) does not seem necessary in this discussion.

Nearly always, the origin of these pains is defined as "benign" because it is attributed to a morphological-mechanical conflict of degenerative origin inside the vertebral canal between bone or disc structures and nerve roots. There are also more selective attributions to the posterior joints ("facet" joints, or "interapophyseal" or "zygapophyseal" joints), to not better localised "tears" or "muscle" spasm, and to not better specified "postural" alterations.

This volume deals with lumbago from a "benign" cause in the lumbosacral spine and excludes other less or much less "benign" causes such as vertebral collapses, fractures, infections, neoplasms, and rheumopathies. Only a brief mention of malformations will be made. It also excludes all non-spinal, abdominal, or thoracic pathologies, which can generate pain in the lumbar area.

On closer inspection, it should be clarified that the adjective "benign" is somewhat optimistic. For individual patients, lumbago can represent not only the source of intense, prolonged and refractory pain but is also a cause of significant disability.

For the community, then, lumbago is a real calamity. It is among the leading causes of work absence in the industrialised world as it typically strikes, and often for a very long time, people between the ages of 30 and 65 and, therefore, in full working age. Nowadays, there is evidence that lumbago is among the leading causes of disability (according to the World Health Organization) worldwide. The picture can be mild or moderate in individual cases, but due to its very high prevalence, the economic consequences are impressive. Work or sports conditions expose the person to loads and gestures that increase the risk of lumbago. This is a very broad topic in occupational, preventive, legal, and sports medicine and will not be addressed here. We will, therefore, talk about a patient whose history does not suggest a strong traumatic or professional causality.

The "Back Pain": a Cold Case

From a scientific point of view, lumbago is anything but simple. The mechanism of pain origin (the pathogenesis or, if one so prefers, the "physiopathology") is not yet fully understood. Not by chance is the term "lumbago" still official, to which the WHO assigns the code 724.2 of the International Classification of Diseases, ICD. The "disease"—the "D" of Disease—is defined purely descriptively by the presence of pain, or as "algia", whether lumbar or sciatic (e.g., sciatic neuralgia). A pathophysiological term is not used. Today, very few diagnoses survive with this type of definition (perhaps headache, dysmenorrhoea, insomnia, and a few others). For example, one no longer speaks of "malignant tertian fever" to define a form of disease from infestation by malarial plasmodium. No one would accept a purely descriptive diagnosis of "ocular pain" from an ophthalmologist, nor a diagnosis of "abdominal pain" from a surgeon.

In our era, which is witnessing gene therapies, stem cell treatments, and deep brain stimulations, "back pain" hides in the back rows, behind the humble appearance of a "minor" pathology. By contrast, it still represents a cold case for Medicine and an open methodological challenge. Solving at least part of the cold case could not only improve the lives of many people and reduce healthcare costs but also offer original ideas to many other areas of Medicine. This has motivated my scientific curiosity for low back pain: a curiosity that has never faded even though, for my almost five decades as a doctor, I have mainly dealt with disability from other much less "benign" causes.

Narrowing the Field

In this volume, I will mainly discuss chronic conditions characterised, if we accept a certain flexibility in interpreting the varied literature, by episodes of daily pain, even if remitting/recurrent during the day, present for at least 6 weeks. However, the typical case presents pain for many months, if not years. Acute conditions will still have their own space for discussion. The term "acute" often indicates both a high pain intensity and a sudden onset. This does not exclude, therefore, that some forms of "acute" low back pain may have a long duration. This ambiguity will be resolved later with another classification of low back pain. Even the less typical cases will find a space for description.

As for treatment, the general criteria that justify macro-categories of conservative therapies will be discussed, with particular attention paid to forms of exercise.

Pharmacological alternatives and the more invasive ones will still receive some mention.

The text consolidates over 40 years of personal reflection, practical experience, and research on this elusive pathology. The aim is not to provide an anatomical and diagnostic manual since there are already many excellent texts of this type but rather to propose a pathophysiological model that explains as much as possible:

1. The different pictures that emerge from clinical observation (the "phenotypes"), looking contradictory despite a common descriptive diagnosis.
2. The rationale of different therapeutic proposals. The enormous variety of therapeutic proposals appears contradictory with respect to the uniqueness of the descriptive diagnosis (if you have to treat "stomach pain", every proposal is good, and the same goes for "back pain").

Borrowing a well-known metaphor, the text does not provide the clinician with fish but wants to teach him how to fish.

Text Style and Instructions for Use

The structure of the text and its style aim to be halfway between a detailed monograph and a real textbook. The volume is born from a didactic intent: it wants to consolidate decades of my teaching on the subject, carried out in countless seminars and conference events and, above all, in countless lessons. These were mostly held at the University of Milan, where I was a full professor of Physical Medicine and Rehabilitation for 18 years. I am now an Honorary Professor. I have taught this subject mainly to residents of the Residency Program in Physical and Rehabilitation Medicine. Still, I must also mention the Program in Neurology, the classes in Medicine and Surgery, and the master's degree courses in Motor Sciences and Physiotherapy.

Some consequences of this approach:

1. The volume represents my personal thoughts. Many scientific references support them, obviously, but I have not worried too much about supporting every sentence with a bibliographic citation, as is typical for publications in classic scientific journals.
2. The discussion assumes that the reader has basic knowledge of spine anatomy (including its nervous content) and basic notions of orthopaedics and neurology. The iconography, therefore, is minimised but is sufficient to facilitate understanding the pathogenetic mechanism I propose.
3. The text aims to promote critical thinking, not to detail this or that therapeutic modality. On the health "market", the proposals, even just for forms of exercise, are countless, appear contradictory to each other, and in many cases are supported by a vast dedicated literature that would be disrespectful to oversimplify.

4. The text is aimed at those—student or professional—who are interested in disciplines of rehabilitative, neurological and neurosurgical, orthopaedic, rheumatological, or even motor science areas. However, considering how widespread and trans-disciplinary this pathology is, I would not exclude general medicine, geriatrics, and pain therapy.

5. The clinical description of typical patients and the semiotic manoeuvres I present do not intend to replace the classic orthopaedic and neurological semiotics nor minimise the obligation of anamnesis and general objective examination. Instead, as will appear evident, the clinical narrative with which I describe "types" of patients aims to highlight symptoms and manoeuvres that will find a rational placement within a unitary pathophysiological model that explains through the "types" themselves the majority of clinical cases: it remains understood that the search for a full understanding of the phenomenon remains an open adventure.

Contents

Part I

Observing the Patient

Lower Back Pain and its Contradictions

I will try to make "lower back pain" more "specific". Table 1.1 illustrates eight contradictions inherent in the common case history of "lower back pain" that I will try to resolve during the discussion.

Table 1.1 shows that, in the face of a single descriptive diagnosis, there can be "phenotypic" and behavioural pictures that are entirely contradictory among themselves, each with respect to the *imaging* diagnostic to which it is associated. I will, therefore, attempt a more precise description of these points. I should thus allow these observations to be framed in a single pathogenetic model (or pathophysiological if you will), which I will arrive at in Chap. 8.

Today, the dominant clinical attitude is to generically frame under the "umbrella" term of lower back pain or lumbosciatica the most diverse patients and to immediately jump to the *imaging* of the lumbosacral spine. The *imaging* often does not explain the clinical picture and does not change, even if the patient's pain changes for better or worse. Therefore, due to excessive trust in technology, a critical phase of the clinical investigation is skipped, which consists of the accurate anamnestic reconstruction and the observation of the patient at the bedside (the classic neurological and orthopaedic semiotics) and during the patient's motor behaviours.

Table 1.1 Contradictions in the different "phenotypes" found in the case history of "lower back pain"

1. Antalgic position flexed or extended
2. The pain increases at rest or with load
3. Discrepancy imaging-symptoms
4. Pain in pregnancy with negative imaging
5. Risk factors: the same cardiovascular ones
6. Spontaneous healing, imaging unchanged
7. Successful curing, imaging unchanged
8. Persistence of clinical improvement, imaging unchanged

© The Author(s), under exclusive license to Springer Nature Switzerland AG 2025
L. Tesio, *Low Back Pain and Sciatica*,
https://doi.org/10.1007/978-3-031-78534-4_1

If clinical observation is not underestimated (which requires method and experience), even apparently similar patients will finally start to appear different. This attention to clinical observation has supported my attempt to construct a pathogenetic model that tries to explain (and not just observe) the different "phenotypic" pictures. I will start from the first contradictory point, the one related to the different antalgic positions preferred by different patients, although all "lower back pain sufferers".

1.1   The Two Main Clinical Types: The Patient with Flexor Relief and the Patient with Extensor Relief

I will define two main phenotypes (or "types" *tout-court*), represented in a simplistic way by Fig. 1.1a and b and which describe how the patient presents or which positions, during the medical examination, alleviate or exacerbate the pain. The two "types" are defined based on the position of the lumbar spine that usually provides relief: the "flexor" patient, widely prevalent, who feels better with a flexed lumbar

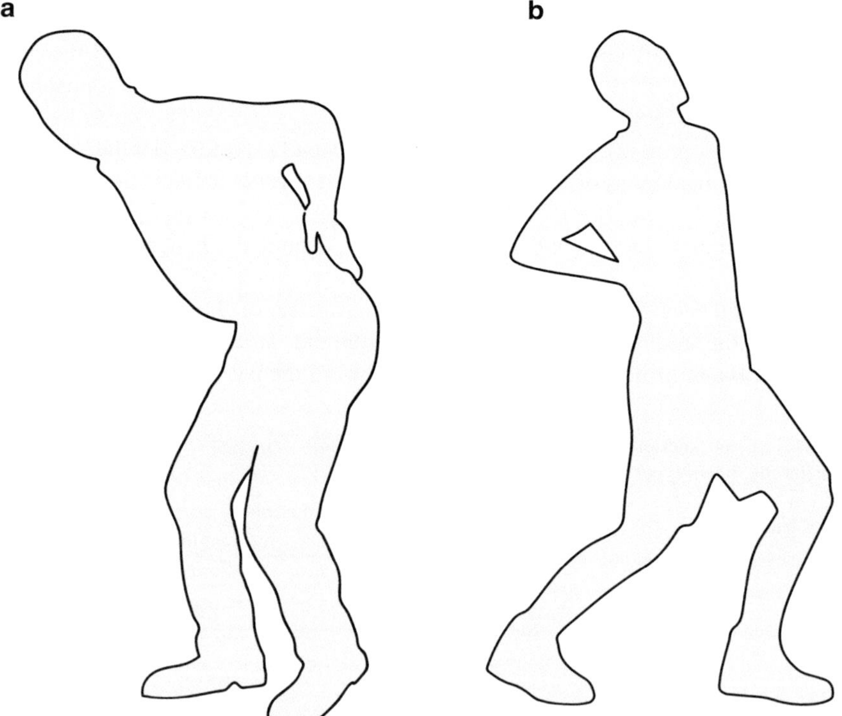

Fig. 1.1 The two main "phenotypes" of low back pain. (**a**) The "flexor" patient: the lumbar or sciatic pain is reduced with the trunk flexed or less extended than usual. (**b**) The "extensor" patient: the lumbar or sciatic pain is reduced with the trunk extended or less flexed than usual

Table 1.2 Dichotomous classification of the two phenotypes of patients suffering from low back pain (lumbosciatica and/or sciatica and/or cruralgia) for at least 6 weeks

Flexor-type patient	Extensor-type patient
The lumbar and sciatic pain appears or increases mainly:	
• With the extension (lordotization) of the lumbar spine • At rest • At night or upon waking • With prolonged trunk positions and their variations	• With the flexion (delordotization) of the lumbar spine • Under load (walking, lifting weights) • During the day • With increased abdominal pressure (Valsalva manoeuvre, cough, sneeze, abdominal pressure) • Both stationary and in any change of trunk position
The pain has intensity:	
• Medium-low	• High
Onset:	
• Gradual (days)	• Sudden or quick (instant; hours)
Predominant qualitative description:	
• Dog bite, cramp, weight, agony	• Sharp pain, burning, electric shock
Neurological signs (many exceptions; however rare):	
• Absent	• Lasègue • Hypoesthesia • Achilles hyporeflexia
Pharmacologically, the pain responds mainly to:	
• NSAIDs	• Steroids (dexamethasone)

Note. The classification is based on the preferred pain-relieving position and the mechanisms that intensify the pain

spine (or at least less extended than usual), and the "extensor" patient, much rarer, who feels better with an extended lumbar spine (or at least straightened). Similarly, the flexor patient may report increased pain if the spine extends, while the extensor patient may report worsening pain if the lumbar spine flexes. As will be seen, the "phenotype" flexor or extensor does not only include the position of the lumbar spine.

A syndromic description, or "how and when the pain intensifies" (the reason that imposes the flexed or extended position), is the object of Table 1.2. The two types described can overlap partly, but it is better to be dichotomous for teaching purposes. In both cases, it should be remembered that I am referring to a patient with daily pain - even if remitting/recurrent during the day - that has lasted for at least 6 weeks but that usually has been present for many months or years and in which fractures, infections, spinal neoplasms have been ruled out (for malformations, see later).

The Flexor-Type Patient: Low Back Pain, Sciatica, Lumbar Radiculopathy

2

Textbooks give a lot of emphasis to the case that is, however, the least common: the acute patient with sciatica and neurological signs, who corresponds to the phenotype that I have defined here as "extensor" because he finds at least partial relief with the extension of the lumbar spine. I will deal with this case after the "flexor" patient, who is much more common. I don't think there are statistics based on this classification. The extensor type might prevail in an emergency room or an orthopaedic clinic because the patient usually presents intense and sudden symptoms. My outpatient experience with several thousand patients suggests that in a physiatric clinic, 95% of the cases arrive in the chronic phase. Therefore, the most common case is from the beginning or has become, over time, of the flexor type. Beware: this means that, given the large numbers typical of this caseload, the extensor patient is also common.

2.1 Medical History

The flexor patient usually (let's say in 80% of cases) is between 40 and 70 years old. Perhaps 20% of cases cover the age ranges 25–40 and 70–90 (but more extreme cases always exist). Men and women are equally represented. Unless (rarely) this is the first medical contact, the patient immediately shows images of nuclear magnetic resonance (MRI) or computed axial tomography (CT) of the spine, often repeated. At least in 50% of cases, an X-ray and an electromyography are also available. As all clinicians know, the patient is anxious to immediately propose his/her interpretation of the problem before even describing it ("I had an MRI, and there's a disc herniation…"). You have to listen to him but only up to a point, even at the cost of disappointing him. You have to ask him to tell the story from the end: that is, from the symptoms. The instrumental outcomes will be considered in light of the medical history and the visit.

© The Author(s), under exclusive license to Springer Nature
Switzerland AG 2025
L. Tesio, *Low Back Pain and Sciatica*,
https://doi.org/10.1007/978-3-031-78534-4_2

2.2   The Pain: Which and Where

The patient reports unilateral, median or bilateral pain in the lumbar area: the pain onset was gradual or acute but without a triggering event. It is possible (although rare) that the patient reports having sustained repeated efforts with the lumbar spine in the weeks or days before the onset: the classic relocation or the strenuous mobilisation of a disabled person. The current episode of pain is usually not the first. In the past, there have been more or less acute episodes, including classic "lumbar blocks" often dubbed "witch's blows". The pain is not such that it critically impairs mobility. It is described with great difficulty, usually as "weight" possibly associated with "stabs", but the paraphrases can be the most varied. If it spreads along the lower limb, the pain is localised to the muscle and typically described as "cramp", "biting dog", "a weight", and more rarely "burning" (see Table 1.2).

2.3   The Temporal and Spatial Distribution of Pain

An essential medical history point is the temporal distribution of current pain. Typically, it is present, or at least intensifies, with prolonged positions: sitting, standing, and even lying down (which often disturbs sleep). The worst moment is the change of position (supine—sitting, sitting—standing, getting out of the car, and similar). Pain is often worse when the patient gets out of bed in the morning.

Pain spreading to the lower limb (in my experience, approximately 50% of cases) can have three characteristic distributions indicative of suffering from different lumbosacral roots in addition to the lumbar area. Let's see them:

- Groin and - in men - the testicle and the medial surface of the thigh; radicular territory L3;
- Anterior and lateral surface of the thigh and leg; territory L4-L5;
- Calf and foot sole; territory L5-S1.

Whatever the distribution, it is also necessary to distinguish referred pain (the most frequent) from radiating pain.

2.3.1   The Distribution: Referred Pain and Radiating Pain

A very didactic synthesis on the subject is present in two relatively recent reviews [1, 2]. By "radiating" pain, we mean pain distributed over a territory corresponding to the sensitive dermatomes, innervated by the sensitive roots, and therefore also defined as "radicular". "Referred" pain is perceived in a location different from the lesion site. It is thus understood how pain caused by a vertebral pathology and localised to the lower limb is always "referred to". The neurophysiological basis of the "reference" is the convergence at the spinal level, on common interneurons, of sensitive fibres that convey painful stimuli from different body sites sharing the metameric origin. The best-known example is perhaps that of pain on the ulnar side of the left hand in the case of myocardial infarction.

The suffering of an interapophyseal joint or a ligament (the posterior longitudinal, a yellow ligament or an interspinous one) can "refer" pain to muscles according to a distribution that is only apparently capricious, well described already 85 years ago [3]. Even meningeal irritation can cause referred pain. The theme becomes a little more complicated in the case of serous membranes (peritoneum, pericardium, pleura, synovia) and, in general, of the viscera. The viscera lose a precise metameric radicular distribution. Consequently, the "reference" of visceral pain, unlike "somatic" pain, can recall multiradicular distributions, even in anatomical locations distant from the current one. For example, in addition to the well-known case of the reference to the hand of pain of myocardial origin, gallbladder pain can generate right subscapular pain [2].

Referred pain, of both somatic and visceral origin, is not associated with radicular signs because there is no direct compression of sensitive or motor roots. In the case of lumbar problems, a distribution on the glutei and thigh is much more frequent than below the knee. The distribution can, therefore, resemble a partial radicular distribution, but it is not identical.

Pain can follow a dermatomeric distribution (radiating pain) if it derives from the suffering of a sensitive root or the corresponding spinal ganglion. The distribution can be partial, but in this case, as a rule, it is only distal, below the knees, and not only proximal (as instead happens for referred pain). Simple compression can induce the spinal ganglion to generate discharges of action potentials that create acute stabbing "electric" pain along the entire course of the corresponding spinal root. The same can happen, for a moment, in case of direct compression of the sensitive root. However, gradual or chronic compression of the sensitive root only generates neurological signs (hypoesthesia, loss of osteotendinous reflexes) but not pain. For pain to appear, there must be an inflammatory process of the root itself [4]. It should be clarified that the term "sciatica" is somewhat imprecise since it tends to define both pain referred to the lower limb and actual radiating-radicular pain. Conversely, the adjective "radicular" is often used to indicate pain of different origin in the lower limb.

From the distinction between the two types of pain, at least four considerations arise:

1. it is understandable why the radiating or radicular pain is much rarer than the referred one
2. Phenomena of "allodynia" (perception of usually non-painful stimuli as painful) are possible only in the case of authentically radicular-radiating pain.
3. The herniated disc often plays a decisive role in causing radicular pain, but - as will be seen later in the discussion - it is much less influential on lumbar or referred pains (which, of course, does not exclude that herniation plays a significant causal role).

4. The different mechanisms of pain explain the well-known observation that disc herniectomy almost always resolves authentic radicular pain but more rarely lumbar or referred sciatic pain.

Therefore, it should be remembered that standard imaging techniques find it difficult to identify a source of "referred" pain. At the same time, they find it much easier to identify causes of pain radiating in a root territory.

2.4   Subjective Description of Pain

The type of pain does not seem to have very reproducible characteristics among different subjects. Instead, the difficulty in describing is expected. The description depends significantly on the patient's linguistic abilities and emotional experience. Very metaphorical descriptions of pain are widespread. For example, as already highlighted, this could be described as "a biting dog", "a cramp", or "burning", rarely as "electric shock". The same applies to its functional impact ("something that doesn't let me work"). Generally, a constant background of pain (in the best case, a "discomfort") with frequent exacerbations is reported. Entirely pain-free days are rare.

2.5   Therapies: Which (Did Not) Work

When the patient meets a specialist after previous visits, he usually already has a history of weeks or months of pain and, therefore, a history of several diagnostic and therapeutic attempts. Often, in previous years, any past episodes had a spontaneous remission or responded temporarily to the most varied treatments that, if replicated, failed. The list of recent attempts during the current episode can be very long, for example:

- drugs: from steroids to NSAIDs to paracetamol, up to medications for neuropathic pain;
- the most varied instrumental physical therapies: various forms of diathermy or deep heating such as short- or micro-waves and ultrasound therapy; neuro-analgesic therapies such as laser therapy and electrotherapies, etc.;
- passive manual therapies: massage, mobilisation and vertebral manipulation according to various methods;
- various techniques of therapeutic exercise;
- more or less invasive "pain therapies": acupuncture, mesotherapy, local or epidural infiltrations, ozone therapy, electrostimulation with epidural electrodes;
- corsets;
- prescription of simple bed rest.

Many of these treatments have induced mild and short-term improvements in the past. In the long term, some efficacy is typically attributed to NSAIDs, which have a reliable but always temporary effect. One or more diverse professionals have been consulted: general practitioner, orthopedist, physiatrist, neurosurgeon (rare: the neurologist and the rheumatologist), physiotherapists, osteopaths, and chiropractors.

2.6   The Diagnostic History

The diagnoses have often been discordant, generic, or, in any case, different. They range from a pure description ("low back pain" or "sciatica", precisely) to very anatomical interpretations such as disc herniation or intervertebral joint disorder, up to more "holistic" interpretations such as "postural disorder."

It is not uncommon for the patient to have already been proposed for surgery: a hypothesis on which the patient seeks confirmation. There may be a history of surgery already performed with unsatisfactory results. The surgery, proposed or even already performed, will be discussed later.

The patient often turns to the Physiatrist (the physician specialist in Physical and Rehabilitation Medicine), who has rarely been the first on the list. However, I believe this figure is gaining popularity. In any case, the typical patient described above is frightened by the continuous failures. He is generally disappointed and distrustful but hopeful in yet another "last resort".[1]

2.7   Pain and Daily Movements

You must ask the right questions and seek consistency between the onset of pain and daily motor activities. Typically, in the flexor patient (who, as seen, is usually chronic), the pain worsens not only with the extension of the spine but, in general, with the maintenance of a prolonged position, even supine.[2] It is essential to ask the patients how long they can sit in a car.

---

[1] *A rare but not exceptional indicator of the patient's distrust of the doctor is the "forgetfulness" of instrumental exams. Contrary to the typical behaviour of the patient who exhibits a plethora of instrumental exams, often repeated unnecessarily at short intervals, there is the behaviour - not exceptional - of the patient who presents, declaring to have forgotten them all. I have no proof of what I claim. Still, I suspect this represents an attempt to "reset" the counter for fear that the umpteenth doctor will uncritically rely on the previous and disappointing results. According to my experience, a clue that a relationship of trust has been established is given by the fact that - at the end of the visit - the patient hurries to propose to transmit or bring in person as soon as possible the "forgotten" exams, hoping for a second round of evaluation with the exams on the table.*

[2] *Why does the pain worsen when the disc pressure decreases, for example, in the supine position and at rest? As widely clarified further, the lordosis/extension of the spine reduces the vertebral canal's transverse section and the conjugation foramina's section. Rest reduces the concomitant muscular activity, which, notoriously, acts as a "pump" that facilitates venous drainage. The pathogenetic model supported here has a fundamental element in epidural venous dilation that*

As counterintuitive as this may seem, walking and careful lifting of loads rarely worsen symptoms (except for cases of occupational disease which I cited in the introduction). It would help to ask the patient what happens when walking uphill and downhill. The mountain lovers will invariably report no pain when going uphill, while they report pain when going downhill (a point to which we will return).[3]

It is essential to understand what happens with sleep: often, the patient reports "not finding the position" to sleep or having frequent awakenings due to pain. The patient prefers to fall asleep on his side with one or both lower limbs flexed at the hip and knee "in the fetal position". He rarely prefers the prone position. Even if the patient sleeps continuously, waking up in the morning is still the worst time. The patient will report feeling stiff, blocked, and struggling to get up ("morning stiffness"). The patient invariably states that bending over the sink and then getting up is a tragedy: afterwards, as he/she moves, the situation improves, only to worsen at the end of the day.

Coughing, sneezing, and abdominal pressure (the classic "Valsalva manoeuvres") can cause momentary exacerbations, but these are not frequent cases.

2.8   Not Just Low Back Pain: Painless Claudication (*claudicatio spinalis*)

2.8.1   The Syndrome of the Narrow Lumbar Canal (Spinal Stenosis)

The patient may report mild to moderate lumbar, sciatic, or crural pain but is mainly affected by a disabling reduction of walking distance. After a particular stretch of road (usually varying between 50 and 500 m), "the legs no longer go". Low back pain appears to be the least of his/her problems. A syndrome of the narrow lumbar canal (*spinal stenosis*) should be suspected. This syndrome deserves separate treatment even if the patient who suffers from it falls into the macro-category of "flexor" patients because he/she prefers an anteflexed trunk position both in static and walking. An anatomical reminder is needed first.

2.8.2   When Is the Canal "Narrow"?

There is no complete agreement on the radiological definition of a "narrow" lumbar canal. One criterion is based on a threshold of the anteroposterior bone diameter of the levels investigated: some propose 13 mm at level L3, and others suggest 11.

---

helps to explain the apparent paradox of a pain of vertebral origin that increases with rest, even when there is a reduction in load on the spine itself.

[3] *Why does downhill walking cause pain and uphill walking does not? In downhill walking, the lumbar spine must remain extended to prevent the body's centre of gravity from projecting outside the base of support. Unless long Nordic walking sticks are used, the patient will experience pain.*

However, the cross-section area and the vertebral canal's overall shape matter. There must be room for the cauda equina roots. If the articular facets invade the canal laterally, the canal assumes the shape of a narrow "isosceles triangle", perhaps leaving the anteroposterior diameter unaffected. An even better definition is that of "cloverleaf shape" (*trefoilness*): the thin "triangle" connects to two lateral interstices that are what remains of the foramina. Unfortunately, the spinal ganglia and roots must pass through these interstices (Fig. 2.1).

2.8.3   History and Characteristics of the Syndrome

The syndrome of spinal stenosis was only defined in the 1950s [5]. The person who suffers from it can be considered a separate case of "flexor patient", affected more by locomotor deficit than by pain. The syndrome often includes, but not necessarily, lumbar pain, sometimes of modest entity, associated or not with modest pains distributed "like short pants". This point must be recalled because it is functional to the construction of the pathogenetic model of lumbosciatic pain that will be proposed here. The patient invariably reports having a reduced walking distance (as a rule, between 50 and 300 m), after which "the legs no longer go" or "they become hard" or "heavy". The patient must stop and possibly sit "crouching" for about 1–3 min, after which he can make the next stretch. Walking, not immobility, generates the problem (contrary to what has been reported so far for the typical flexor patient).

So, the problem is mainly motor. There is a *spinal claudication* [6] often confused with a claudication from vascular pathology, which instead announces itself with acute pains in the calves (in these cases, the arterial circulation is so much more precarious the more distal the segment to be vascularised). The patient typically has performed useless Doppler exams of the lower limbs. The pathophysiology is known, even if neurophysiological alterations have never been demonstrated.[4] The lumbar canal presents a section pathologically narrowed due to osteophytes and hypertrophy of the facets (acquired stenosis), possibly aggravated by concomitant disc protrusions. Rarely is there a congenital alteration or the shortness of the vertebral peduncles (a typical condition in the rare achondroplastic dwarfism). During walking, large nerve trunks come into activity and require high oxygen consumption: the stenosis hinders the radicular circulation, predominantly venous (a point on which we will return), so a classic reversible nerve conduction block is determined. The trunk flexion enlarges the section of the vertebral canal and the conjugation foramina so that the walk can resume. The syndrome can rarely be unilateral.

Some defined this syndrome as "shop windows disease". Many patients at the end of the allowed walking distance must flex the trunk. If they do not have a bench available, they must "bend on their legs", offering an embarrassing image of severe discomfort. For this reason, "they pretend to look at a shop window". As rare as it is

---

[4] *Transient alterations of the F wave should be observed due to the multi-radicular motor conduction block. However, no specific alterations have ever been evidenced at rest, and studying the F wave while walking is practically impossible.*

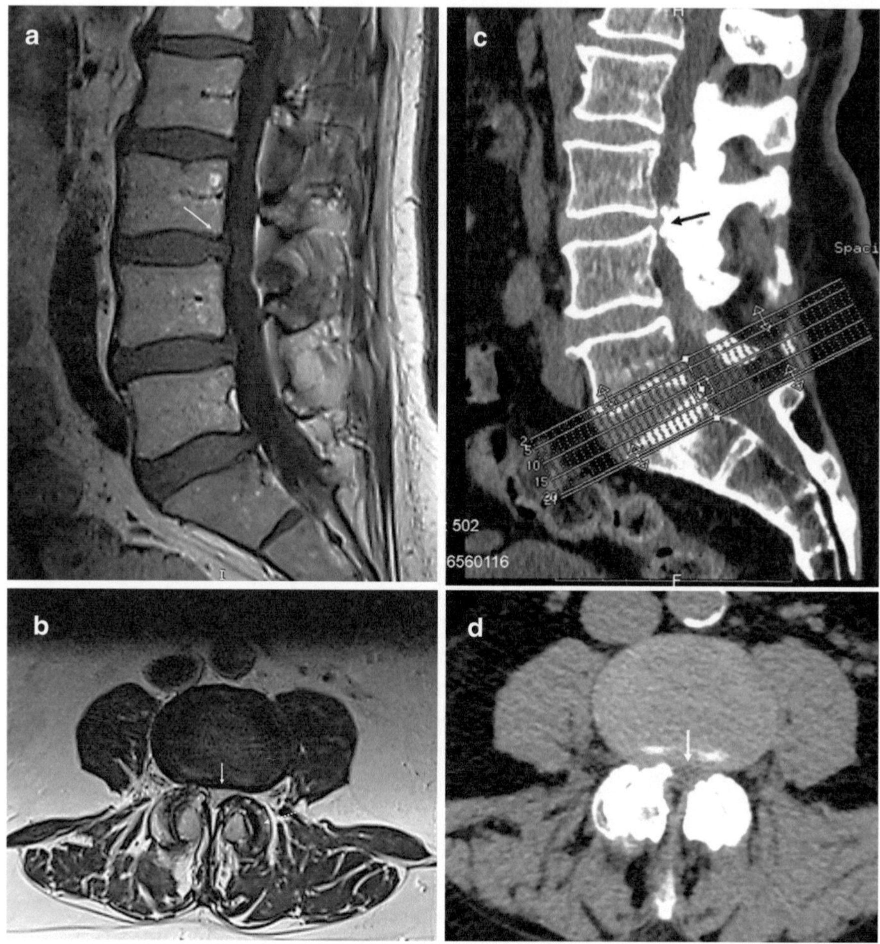

Fig. 2.1 Images of a severely narrowed "cloverleaf" lumbar canal. 75-year-old man. Walking distance is limited to 200 m. Weakness of the plantar flexors and pronator muscles of the foot, with EMG evidence of chronic L5-S1 radicular suffering. There is no low back pain or pain in the lower limbs. In (**a** and **b**): MRI image of the L3-L4 level. In the sagittal section (**a**), only a modest disk protrusion (arrow) is noticeable. In (**b**) (axial section), a significant "cloverleaf" stenosis is noticeable. The continuous arrow indicates the vertebral canal; the arrowhead rests on the modest disk protrusion, barely recognisable for the darker black colour compared to the vertebral body above. The joint effusion between the "facets" constituting the interapophyseal joint is well highlighted (dashed arrow). CT images were taken at the same L3-L4 level in (**c**) and (**d**). Unlike the MRI; the CT scan can highlight marked posterior osteophytosis (black arrow), as it is susceptible to bone mineral density. In (**d**) in the axial section, the narrowed lumbar canal and the disk protrusion (on which the arrow's head rests) are noticeable. The edge of the vertebral plate is well recognisable by its white colour. Unlike the MRI, the CT scan highlights the bone-disk margin better but does not give good evidence of intra-articular effusion between the facets (personal observation)

in this specific manifestation, the term is very evocative of the patients' adaptation strategy. Often, they make well-planned external routes because they are scattered with benches or shop windows at the proper distances.

In the syndrome of the narrow canal, there can be intense lumbar pains at night when there is latent heart failure: it is the "Vesper's curse" on which we will return [7].

It should be noted that stenosis is more frequent at levels L3 and L2, while disc herniation is more frequent at levels L4-L5 and L5-S1. Therefore, the stenosis might be overlooked if only the L3-S1 segments are investigated with CT or MRI. The prognosis and conservative therapy of this syndrome will be discussed in a dedicated paragraph.

2.8.4   Two Syndromes or One? Stenosis and "Restless" Legs

For reasons that will be clarified later, there is a strong suspicion that stenosis can interfere with sleep, causing nocturnal awakenings due to the "restless legs syndrome". Sir Thomas Willis, who described the eponymous cerebral arterial anastomotic circle, described this syndrome in 1672. However, the most popular name is due to the Swedish neurologist Karl-Axel Ekbom, who coined it in 1944 [8]. This condition is also called Willis-Ekbom disease.

The "syndrome" is quite common (percentages are reported close to 10% of adults – mostly beyond age 60, in my experience) and has at least three typical characteristics:

- it is present at night and causes awakening;
- it causes an urgent desire to move the lower limbs;
- the disturbance is alleviated by movement (especially by walking).

For the diagnosis, it is necessary first to exclude cramp-like disorders or other movement disorders (for example, tics or epilepsy). Until today, a "central" neurological diagnosis prevails, which makes it a movement disorder related to dystonias or tremors. The syndrome is quite common in Parkinson's disease and can respond to dopaminergic drugs. Metabolic causes and co-causes have also been hypothesised: iron, magnesium and selenium deficiency, and hyperthyroidism, but without clear experimental evidence. In truth, none of these explanations is entirely convincing.

The disorder is often associated with pregnancy and a narrow lumbar canal. Patients with Parkinson's disease notoriously have significant postural problems of the spine [9], and the symptomatic effectiveness of dopaminergic drugs is not conclusive about the diagnosis. It seems reasonable, therefore, to hypothesise that this "disease" may also be a manifestation of ischemia of the cauda equina from compression and venous stasis, at least in a good percentage of cases (see below about this hypothesis).

2.9   Considering Instrumental Examinations

I prefer to proceed to the clinical examination before evaluating instrumental findings and reports during a visit. However, this would somewhat disappoint a patient who has spent time and money on these exams and has built his explanation of the problem based on them. In ascending order, I consider X-ray, CT, and MRI essential. The radiography (which I rarely request) can be, at most, a good complement. In any case, except for glaring cases, no imaging examination is probative of a causal relationship with the pain.

MRI or CT usually reveal reasons for radicular compression: hernia or disc protrusion, single or on multiple levels; osteophytes. The finding of joint emission of two contiguous homolateral roots from a single conjugation foramen (*conjoint roots*) is rare [10]. Another rare finding should be mentioned: the stacking of the roots due to their excessive length (*redundant roots*) [11].

Idiopathic scoliosis (a potential source of joint or disc alterations) is better observed with an X-ray. A spondylolisthesis is better observed with MRI or X-ray. Rare malformations (for example, metameric differentiation defects, hemivertebrae, synostosis) are more easily noticeable with X-rays (it's better to have oblique projections). Bone details (thus, osteophytes and the verbal-discal border) are better observed with CT, but you need to know which levels to focus the examination on (which gives horizontal sections, and the sagittal and frontal planes only offer reconstructed images). For the spondylolysis (usually well visible with oblique X-ray projections), the CT must be performed with knowledge of the diagnostic question because the orientation of the "cut" of the CT images must be specific (see the dedicated paragraph in the Appendix).

As a rule, MRI or CT show alterations compatible with the patient's symptoms but not probative. Defining a disc alteration as a protrusion (*bulging*) or hernia is often a purely linguistic question. There are no standard parameters to choose one of the two terms. However, the definition of extruded (or expelled) hernia is much more precise: the disc material has lost continuity with the original disc. It can migrate laterally and vertically (Figs. 2.1a, b, and d). One should keep in mind, however, that disc protrusion is very common even in entirely asymptomatic patients (approximately 40% of cases). One or more protrusions, even marked, of the lumbar discs, are, therefore, a "normal" finding in the statistical sense of the term.

2.9.1   The Electromyographic Examination: Rarely Necessary

The EMG exam (an acronym for electroneurography/electromyography) is overrated in the case of lumbosciatic pain, and yet it is prescribed very often. I believe that it is at least in part a form of pre-surgical defensive medicine (pre-existing radicular suffering is seen as justifying any therapeutic failures). More generally, the EMG is prescribed simply for its "technological" charm and for the impression of objectivity that patients and not a few doctors report. In reality, the exam is very operator-dependent. In particular, in cases of low back pain, even with pain spreading to the lower limbs, the exam hardly ever brings valuable information for clinical decisions.

Consider that a subject with low back pain (but in reality, anyone over 50 years old) always has subclinical suffering of the lumbosacral nerve roots. Inevitably, the needle exam shows some rare fibrillation potential (expression of recent denervation), a remodelling of the motor units (polyphasic and with increased duration), an expression of reinnervation. This applies to whatever muscles are investigated, all innervated by several lumbar and sacral roots; for example:

- common extensor of the toes and gastrocnemius in case of L5-S1 suffering;
- quadriceps femoris in case of L3-L4 suffering;
- iliopsoas and adductor muscles in case of L2-L3 suffering.

The study of sensory conduction is usually negative, even in sensation loss. Radicular suffering implies damage uphill the ganglion; therefore, the fibres downhill the ganglion, outside the spinal canal, remain intact). If the sensory conduction is altered, we are in either peripheral neuropathy (as a rule, irrelevant for lumbosciatalgia) or nerve compression outside the spine that requires a specific diagnosis.

In the case of long-standing radicular suffering, the motor nerve conduction may show a decrease in the amplitude of the muscle potentials, with slightly reduced conduction speed (a few fast fibres are enough to preserve the minimal latency of the potential's appearance on the muscle). Nothing emerges from the EMG that makes the pain "objective" or legitimises a surgical indication on this basis (even if alternative diagnoses that require surgery may arise by chance). However, I will return later on the differential diagnosis.

Let's now imagine that no data justify the suspicion of non-benign pathologies, so that we can continue the discussion.

2.10   The Objective Clinical Examination

I am referring here to the examination specifically aimed at defining the mechanism (the pathogenesis) that causes the symptoms reported by the patient.

It should be recalled that the context discussed here is still that of a medical visit; therefore, the doctor is not exempt from considering more general clinical observations, including incidental but essential findings for the patient's health.

2.10.1 Segmental Examination at the Bedside

The bedside examination, as a rule, is very disappointing. Inspection and direct palpation of the spine do not provide information. Only rarely does sacroiliac or paravertebral compression between the iliac crest and spinous processes cause pain. The same applies to the compression of the classic Valleix points (where we expect to compress and stretch the sciatic nerve) along the buttock and thigh.

The classic Lasègue sign is rare.[5] As a rule, no sensory or motor neurological signs are found.[6] If there are sensory deficits, these are consistent, on the side of the pain, with a classic mono- or multi-radicular distribution (L3-L4 on the thigh and anteromedial face of the leg, L5-S1 on the lateral face of the leg and laterally to the calf and the posterior face of the thigh, etc.). Typically, the deficit only concerns touch, pain and temperature and does not involve vibratory or kinesthetic sensitivity. In the flexor patient (but also in the extensor, as we will see later), the abduction of the hips against resistance can evoke lumbar pain bilaterally or from the most involved side. Rarely does the same apply to the abdominal contraction, which is easily obtained by asking the patient to lift both[7] lower limbs (i.e., flex the hips) with the legs extended.

On the side of the pain, the Achilles reflex may be dimmed or abolished. The Achilles reflexes are sometimes dimmed bilaterally, even without other radicular signs, as can happen in normal conditions. Hardly tendon areflexia or hyporeflexia can be found.

If so, findings should suggest radicular damage; usually, however, this finding demonstrates a spinal algogenic inhibition of the tendon reflex (also bilaterally). The reflex can quickly reappear as soon as the pain is resolved. More rarely, the same phenomenon affects the patellar reflex. Incidentally, hypoesthesia can also reappear when the pain disappears, as it can also represent a central inhibitory

---

[5] *The Lasègue sign consists of passive flexion of the knee and hip and subsequent extension of the knee. An entirely equivalent version is called the "straight leg raising test" (lifting the lower limb with the leg extended). The manoeuvre is positive if it generates pain radiating to the posterior face of the thigh and leg within 45° of lifting. The manoeuvre stretches the sciatic nerve, indicating radicular suffering (L5 and S1). However, it must be excluded that the pain is simply due to the stretching of shortened hamstring muscles, a frequent finding in a sedentary population. If the pain is neurogenic, it likely arises from stretching the dural sheath, accompanying the sensitive and motor roots at their emergence from the conjugation foramen. Consequently, Lasègue is a sign of meningeal irritation, so much so that the same manoeuvre is called the Kernig sign in the clinical diagnosis of meningitis. The dural sac can also stretch by flexing the head (Brudzinski sign). I will return to meningeal pain later.*

[6] *A paragraph will be dedicated to strength deficits (very rare in this type of patient) and some additional notes on sensory deficits in the two types of patients, flexor and extensor.*

[7] *Lifting only one lower limb requires almost no abdominal contraction. The gesture involves stabilisation of the pelvis, which would otherwise rotate forward (anteversion), "pulled" by the iliac and rectus femoris muscles. If shortened, these muscles should lose force. The large contralateral gluteus plays the primary role of retroversion stabiliser if only one lower limb is lifted. By contrast, retroversion can only be performed by the abdominals (especially the rectus) if both lower limbs are lifted. The moment determined by the weight of the lower limbs is more remarkable the longer their lever arm; consequently, a higher effort is required to keep the limbs lifted with the legs extended for a few degrees relative to the bed than in a more flexed position at both the hip and the knee. Forced hip abduction has the medium gluteus and tensor fasciae latae muscles as primary agonists. The manoeuvre should be performed on one side at a time. The abductor muscles "pull" the iliac bone towards the trochanter. Therefore, a stabilising contraction of the homolateral quadratus lumborum is needed, which, however, compresses the first three lumbar vertebrae laterally and creates an overall lumbar concavity: this reduces the diameter of the conjugation foramina from which the lumbar roots emerge.*

phenomenon with an analgesic function (anaesthesia for analgesic purposes). We will return to this point in Chap. 8.

At this point, one should check whether the pain can be evoked, or at least worsened, with a simple extension manoeuvre or, to use another term, by enhancing the lumbar spine's lordosis. The patient remains supine but has flexed legs that protrude from the foot edge of the bed.[8] As a rule, a shortening of the ileo-psoas and rectus femoris (a frequent phenomenon in a sedentary population) in this manoeuvre causes pelvis anteversion and enhanced lumbar spine lordosis. The examiner can further accentuate the lumbar extension by trying to insert his forearm under the lumbar spine; if the forearm passes, there is excessive lordosis. Not surprisingly, the pain - whether lumbar or sciatic - often appears or intensifies.

Inspection and, in particular, spine palpation usually do not provide any relevant information. No typical "trigger points" [12] are identified. The classic Manual Medicine codified by Robert Maigne [13] greatly emphasises the search for skin signs (see below) that reveal sympathetic hyperactivity. These may confirm the organic nature of the disorder and guide on the vertebral segment involved even in the absence of radicular signs familiar to neurology (hypoesthesia, weakness, abolition of osteotendinous reflexes). These latter signs depend on the suffering of fibres that pass through the anterior branch of the spinal nerve (the nerve that originates from the confluence of the motor and sensitive roots at the exit from the conjugation foramen) and are directed to the limbs. Instead, the signs evoked by palpation of the spine derive from the suffering of orthosympathetic branches attached to the posterior branch of the spinal nerve. They are part of the syndrome Maigne defined as "minor intervertebral disorder". Let us cite here pain elicited with the "pinching-rolling" of the skin, the presence of areas of skin "like orange peel", and increased dermographism (excessive redness in intensity, spread and duration to digital pressure) with a nearly radicular distribution. In any case, It is doubtful that any radicular signs will be found in these patients.

2.10.2 Behavioural Motor Examination

Postural changes (supine/standing/sitting) can accentuate the pain; statics in itself do not. Typically, trunk flexion (as far as it is allowed without causing painful stretching of the hamstring muscles) does not generate further pain; in fact, it can alleviate it because, as will be clarified later, a reduced lordosis and by greater force flexion (or kyphosis if you will) of the lumbar spine decompresses the spinal roots. The opposite happens for trunk extension, mainly when associated with trunk

---

⁸*The manoeuvre is also known as the Wasserman sign, analogous to the Lasègue sign, as it stretches the spinal roots (in this case, L3 and L4). Regarding the meningeal nature of the sign, the same applies as reported in the previous note on the Lasègue sign. However, a significant difference lies in the fact that in the Wasserman, contrary to what happens in the Lasègue, the lumbar spine is easily lordotic (directly from the stretching of the psoas and indirectly from the anteversion of the pelvis caused by the stretching of the iliacus and rectus femoris muscles). The lordosis can generate pain due to direct root compression for anatomical reasons, which will be clarified later.*

rotation towards the painful side in cases where the symptoms are lateralised. If the patient is supine, it is easier for him to rotate the pelvis. If he spins it towards the non-painful side, it effectively generates a twist of the lumbar spine towards the painful side.

Walking usually does not cause problems. However, if the pain is very lateralised, the load on the painful limb can induce or accentuate the pain. In this case (relatively rare), there may be claudication to escape from support on the affected side, with the trunk inclining towards the opposite side during single support, a gesture similar to the well-known Trendelenburg sign[9] but with a different meaning.

2.10.3 Clinical Evaluation of Imaging Exams of the Lumbosacral Spine

The most reasonable pathogenetic hypothesis, in front of the clinical case described above, is pain from compression on algogenic structures within the vertebral canal at the level of one or more lumbar roots or the first sacral root (S1). Today, this hypothesis is easily supported by MRI or CT images. What do radiological exams related to the lumbosacral spine typically report? These reports are pretty variable in describing the situation. As a rule, as already mentioned, the reports highlight degenerative joint phenomena: osteophytes generated by the interapophyseal joints (or "facet" joints"), narrowed canal, which will be discussed later, moderate antero- or rarely retro-listhesis, hypertrophy of the yellow ligaments (which connect the laminae of the adjacent vertebral arches).[10] The real protagonist of the reports, usually, is the presence of disc prolapses of various degrees: modest disc protrusions (bulging), frank protrusions or hernias; rarely, hernias are extruded.

No rule defines a disc prolapse as a protrusion or hernia based on size (Fig. 2.2). Conversely, we speak of an extruded hernia only when fragments of the nucleus pulposus have escaped from an annulus fibrosus torn, and rarely are they found

---

[9] *The interpretation is not analogous to that which applies to the authentic Trendelenburg sign. This consists of the lateral "fall" of the pelvis towards the side in suspension due to insufficient abductor moment of the supporting hip (for various muscular, nervous or osteoarticular reasons)—the trunk balances by bending towards the supporting side, generating lumbar concavity. In the case of lumbar sciatica, the lateral flexion of the trunk (associated with lumbar concavity) occurs towards the lower limb of the unaffected side when it is in suspension and is primitive, not compensatory for a pelvic abduction failure. Its purpose is to attenuate, during the load on the supporting limb, the radicular compression, laterally flexing the lumbar column towards the opposite side, thus creating on the painful side a lumbar convexity that dilates the foramina of conjugation. Typically, using a stick on the healthy side, rested on the ground when the affected limb loads, reduces or nullifies the true Trendelenburg. On the contrary, the inclination in the case of sciatica is a pain-relieving behaviour already compensatory in itself, and the stick, from whichever side it is carried, does not prevent the movement.*

[10] *A clarification: the Greek term "olísthesis" means "slippage". The initial Greek omega, endowed in this word with a particular superscript sign called "soft spirit", is omitted in English (and other languages). So, speaking of "listhesis" and not "olisthesis" is correct.*

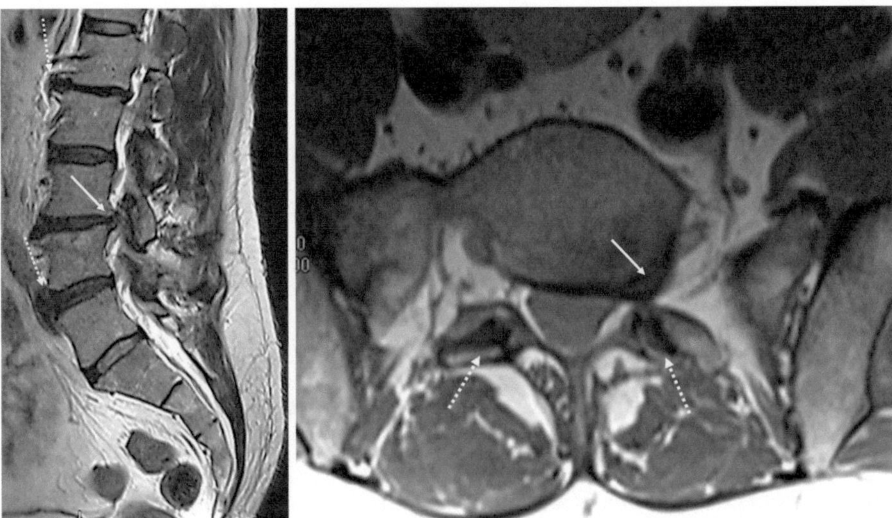

Fig. 2.2 Disc herniations. A 45-year-old man has been suffering from left lumbosciatica for 8 months without radicular signs. MRI images. It should be remembered that the axial (horizontal) images in MRI (and also in CT) are "viewed from below": the left side is to the right of the observer. In the image on the left, giving the sagittal section, a hernia of the third lumbar disc (continuous white arrow) is recognisable in the vertebral canal. The first four lumbar discs are completely dehydrated (between the first and second lumbar vertebra, there is a picture of a "black disc") or partially (second, third and fourth disc). At the L1-L2 level in front of the vertebral bodies, osteophytes are noticeable, and a disk protrusion is also evident between the fourth and fifth lumbar vertebra (dashed white arrow). Anterior osteophytes are entirely asymptomatic. In the image on the right: axial section at level L5-S1. An intraforaminal hernia on the left side is noticeable (continuous white arrow). The interapophyseal joints appear moderately hypertrophic, with a relevant internal effusion (dashed white arrows) (personal observation)

cranially or caudally with respect to the segment from which they emerge after they have detached the posterior longitudinal ligament.

The position of the protrusion or hernia is essential. This could be median, lateralised, or even more lateralised (Fig. 2.2 on the right) to penetrate the already crowded conjugation foramen from which the spinal roots emerge. It is less frequent that the protrusion or hernia is bilateral. The exit from the vertebral canal is rare but not exceptional. In this case, the protrusion or hernia is described as extra-foraminal. Exceptional (and usually post-traumatic) is the case of a hernia that comes to acutely compress more roots of the *cauda equina* or even the spinal cone, causing immediate flaccid paraplegia, but this is, obviously, a surgical emergency quite different from the situation we are dealing with here.

2.10.4 (In)congruence Between Anamnesis, Neuromotor Examination and Imaging

Degenerative pictures like those described above are widespread also in people who do not suffer from low back pain or in people (quite fortunate) who have never suffered. On the other hand, the same images can be associated with symptoms and signs of varying severity, a phenomenon that has generated many pathogenetic models supported by little evidence. To clarify the issue, we had to wait for the description of the disc hernia by Mixter and Barr in 1934 [14] and, in practice, the advent of CT and MRI several decades later.

2.10.5 Why There Can Be a Contradiction Between Imaging and Clinical Picture

This apparent contradiction is among the most important that a rational pathogenesis model must resolve. It should be remembered that lumbosciatic pain, according to the model mentioned here, always has a mechanical origin within the vertebral canal. However, two very tenacious beliefs must be countered:

1. Sciatica should be a primarily inflammatory process of the nerve root, peripheral nerve, or even primarily of the muscle that reacts with a painful "contraction" to climate changes or mechanical efforts. This leads to the frequent use of both B-complex multivitamin drugs, which find a solid neurological indication only in peripheral neuropathies caused by nutritional deficiency, and the use of muscle relaxants, for which the evidence of efficacy is at least nebulous,
2. A disc herniation would be ruled out if no neurological signs exist. If there is no loss of sensitivity or strength, tendon hyporeflexia, positive Lasègue sign within 45°, or Wasserman sign, the presence of a disc herniation among the causes of pain should be excluded.

These two beliefs survive (it must be reiterated: tenaciously) from a time much earlier than the year 1934 in which the scientific community recognised the disc herniation as a nosological entity (although possible precursors of Mixter and Barr are emerging) [15]. Until then, the gelatinous material found in the epidural space, evident in many autopsies, was considered a benign "chondroma". Cervical pain, low back pain, and sciatica, without other objective findings and considering the frequent spontaneous resolution of pain, were interpreted as nonspecific inflammatory diseases of the nerve or muscle ("I caught a cold breeze…"). In a historical study conducted on a corpse, Mixter and Barr associated the protrusion of the nucleus pulposus of a cervical disc to a case of tetraplegia from spinal compression [14]. Mixter and Barr's observation then extended to cases *post-mortem* that had suffered from severe sciatica even with radicular signs.

The diagnosis *in vivo* became possible with the advent of myelography: contrast fluid was injected inside the dural sac, and the bed on which the patient lay was rotated. Images of *minus* in the diffusion of the contrast fluid revealed the presence of disc herniation, which was eventually found to be quite common. However, myelography was an invasive examination, not without risks, when liposoluble contrast fluids, discovered in 1922, were used. A feared complication was inflammation or arachnoiditis that incarcerated the roots of the cauda equina, creating chronic and intractable pains. Since myelography was an invasive examination, it was usually requested, as a rule, in the presence of a strong suspicion of disc herniation due to clear radicular signs. Much less risky water-soluble contrast fluids were discovered in 1956, but the examination remained invasive [16]. Myelography was almost always confirmatory and, as a rule, suggested the presence and the location of a herniation. From this, the methodological error of believing that a disc herniation was not in play without radicular signs was derived. Other factors had to be invoked (muscle contractions, spinal imbalances, "neuritis", and the like). From the 1980s, CT scans, first, and MRI, later, became widespread, significantly superior to myelography in highlighting disc herniations and their relationship with bone structures. The hypothesis that a disc herniation was present only in the case of frank radicular signs was soon disproved by the frequent finding of disc herniations in low back pain without radicular signs and even in many painless subjects.

As mentioned above, since the neuromotor examination is often silent or little symptomatic, the examiner must look for consistency across findings, especially between the pathological picture shown in the images (it doesn't matter if it's disc degeneration or osteoarthritis) and the leading site of pain. A pain localised to one side will be consistent with a disk protrusion or osteophytosis of the posterior joints on the same side.

References

1. Bogduk N. On the definitions and physiology of back pain, referred pain, and radicular pain. Pain. 2009;147:17–9.
2. Woessner J. Referred pain vs. origin of pain pathology. Pract Pain Manag. 2011; 3(6):1–17.
3. Kellgren JH. A preliminary account of referred pains arising from muscle. BMJ. 1938;1(4023):325–7.
4. Howe JF, Loeser JD, Calvin William H. Mechanosensitivity of dorsal root ganglia and chronically injured axons: a physiological basis for the radicular pain of nerve root compression. Pain. 1977;3:25–41.
5. Verbiest H. A radicular syndrome from developmental narrowing of the lumbar vertebral canal. J Bone Joint Surg. 1954;36B(2):230–7.
6. Evans JG. Neurogenic intermittent claudication. BMJ. 1964;2:985–7.
7. LaBan M. "Vespers curse" night pain. The bane of hypnos. Arch Phys Med Rehabil. 1984;65:501–4.
8. Teive HAG, Munhoz RP, Barbosa ER. Professor Karl-Axel Ekbom and restless legs syndrome. Parkinsonism Relat Disord. 2009;15:254–7.
9. Galbusera F, Bassani T, Stucovitz E, Martini C, Ismael Aguirre MF, Berjano PL, et al. Surgical treatment of spinal disorders in Parkinson's disease. Eur Spine J. 2018;27:101–8.
10. Cannon B, Hunter S, Picaza J. Nerve-root anomaly in lumbar-disc surgery. J Neurosurg. 1962;19(3):208–14.

11. Yang SM, Park HK, Cho SJ, Chang JC. Redundant nerve roots of cauda equina mimicking intradural disc herniation: a case report. Korean J Spine. 2013;10(1):41–3.
12. Travell JG, Simons DG, Donnelly JM. Dolore e disfunzioni miofasciali. Manuale per i trigger point. Padova: Piccin Nuova Libraria; 2020.
13. Maigne R. Dolori di origine vertebrale. Comprendere, diagnosticare e trattare. New York: Elsevier; 2009.
14. Mixter WJ, Barr JS. Rupture of the intervertebral disc with involvement of the spinal canal. N Engl J Med. 1934;211(5):210–5.
15. Stienen MN, Surbeck W, Tröhler U, Hildebrandt G. Little-known Swiss contributions to the description, diagnosis, and surgery of lumbar disc disease before the Mixter and Barr era: Historical vignette. J Neurosurg Spine. 2013;19(6):767–73.
16. Zamora CA, Castillo M. Historical perspective of imaging contrast agents. Magn Reson Imaging Clin N Am. 2017;25(4):685–96.

The Extensor-Type Patient: Typical Clinical Picture

3

The typical "extensor" patient is the one who suffers from the classic "witch's blow". The pain arises acutely at the lumbar and/or sciatic level with radicular or similar-radicular distribution (rarely on the front of the thigh). The picture can have dramatic aspects due to high suffering. This patient hardly ever immediately accesses a specialist referral: a decision entailing waiting times and a painful transfer from home. Often, the patient requests a home visit from their family doctor or presents in the emergency room. The anamnesis is rarely informative.

Every patient tries to give an explanation based on some effort or particular trauma, but as a rule, there is no mechanical event that justifies the onset of pain. Typically, the patient presents an intense paravertebral contraction, stands with the lumbar spine erect or extended and avoids any spine movement. There are no positions that substantially alleviate the symptoms. Coughing, sneezing, and abdominal pressure (the "Valsalva" manoeuvre in general) exacerbate the pain.

There may be vegetative signs: pallor, "cold" sweating (indices of orthosympathetic-adrenergic activation), and nausea. Above all, the popular Lasègue sign (passive flexion of the thigh followed by passive knee extension) is ubiquitous, positive already for 20–30° of lower limb elevation (in the fully equivalent "straight leg raising test, the knee is kept extended from the beginning of the test) There may be associated "referred" hypoesthesia with pseudo-radicular distribution (never very clear), Achilles and patellar hyporeflexia, loss of strength in dorsal or more rarely plantar flexion of the big toe or all the toes of the foot. The lumbar pain is constant, and the pain referred to the lower limb can change with rather unpredictable positions of the lower limbs. Common analgesic anti inflammatory drugs (including NSAIDs) do not work, as well. The same holds for drugs for neuropathic pain. Conversely, opioid drugs can work and - even better - a robust dose of steroids can (I will return to this point). Exceptionally (according to my experience), the patient

© The Author(s), under exclusive license to Springer Nature Switzerland AG 2025

L. Tesio, *Low Back Pain and Sciatica*,
https://doi.org/10.1007/978-3-031-78534-4_3

presents the rigid criteria for treatment with spinal manipulation,[1] which can be successful.

The "extensor" patient is, therefore, the most represented in the classical teaching of these syndromes since he/she often presents the canonical radicular signs but, in reality, is decidedly rare. The hyper-acute picture usually resolves completely and spontaneously within 2–7 days. If the pain subsides and the Lasègue sign disappears, sensation, reflexes, and strength can reappear (I will return to this point). After a few days, the dramatic extensor picture cannot infrequently transform into the more common and tolerable "flexor" picture. In the patient's history, there may be several episodes of "witch's blow", sometimes repeated at intervals of many years and interspersed with long periods without symptoms.

---

[1] The topic of Manual Medicine goes beyond the limits of this book. It can be mentioned here that one of the fundamental criteria for the manipulative manoeuvre requires that the patient has at least one direction of movement of the lumbar spine "free" from pain (a very rare event in these cases): the classic manipulative manoeuvre (thrust), accompanied or not by the typical "crack", accentuates the movement in this direction and can be liberating, for reasons not entirely known. Presumably, the manoeuvre works through a neurophysiological mechanism of releasing pathologically contracted paravertebral muscles in response to pain or to release a synovial and cartilaginous fragment trapped between the facets (see Appendix). The semiology and the execution technique require specific experience. It is a procedure of exclusive medical competence.

Part II

The Foundations of Lumbosciatic Pain

Neurology of Lumbosciatic Pain

4

4.1 Where Are the Pain Receptors? An Anatomical Reminder

Among the most explicit descriptions of the "neurology of lower back pain", I must mention those of Nikolai Bogduk [1], Barry Wyke [2] and John W. Frymoyer [3].

Anatomical studies on the subject only agree on some things. For example, Wyke denies that the synovia of the interapophyseal joints and the annulus fibrosus include pain-generating (algogenic) nerve endings, while other authors describe them. In particular, I have not found specific references for the interapophyseal synovia. Still, there is absolute evidence that, in general, the synovial tissue contains algogenic terminations, which makes it unlikely that synovial innervation is lacking only in the posterior vertebral joints [4]. Note that there are also divergent positions on ligamentous anatomy. For example, some argue that no real periosteal tissue is inside the vertebral canal, while other authors describe it.

Therefore, I propose a reasonable synthesis of innervation based on the evidence in the literature.

The following anatomical structures are provided with algogenic nerve endings (non-myelinated fibres, with a diameter of less than 5 microns) involved in nociceptive type pain:

1. discal fibrous annulus;
2. posterior longitudinal ligament;
3. periosteum;
4. epidural fat;
5. vessel walls;
6. dura mater (or dural sac), in ventral portion and radicular sheaths;
7. synovia of the interapophyseal joints;
8. joint capsules and posterior ligaments;
9. muscles (for example, the small interspinous and interapophyseal muscles);
10. cortical and bone marrow.

© The Author(s), under exclusive license to Springer Nature Switzerland AG 2025

L. Tesio, *Low Back Pain and Sciatica*, https://doi.org/10.1007/978-3-031-78534-4_4

It is interesting to note which structures are *not* provided with painful terminations or that, according to the authors, appear to be provided with very scarce terminations:

1. anterior longitudinal ligament;
2. discal "nucleus pulposus";
3. yellow ligaments (or interlaminar ligaments)[1];
4. dura mater, dorsal portion.[2]

The following nerve structures can generate "neuropathic" pain:

1. spinal ganglia;
2. sensitive nerve roots (in case of acute and transitory compression or inflammation).

4.1.1   The Spinal Nerve

The course of the spinal nerve, which is generated by the merging of the sensory and motor roots upon exiting the vertebral canal, deserves special mention. The nerve branches out a lot, but the discussion can be simplified by distinguishing an anterior and a posterior branch. The anterior one merges into the lumbar and sacral plexuses and then into the "long" nerves, subtending the traditional neurological semiotics (femoral nerve, sciatic nerve, etc.). The posterior branch innervates the posterior joints (the "facets") and the paravertebral muscle compartments. Consequently, a disc herniation can cause lower back pain as a form of radiation from the posterior longitudinal ligament and the dural sac and compression of inflamed roots (for the fibres that will merge into the posterior branch of the spinal nerve). I will return to lumbar muscle pain shortly.

4.1.2   The Mechanisms of Pain: "traditional" Compressive Pathogenesis

Except for the rare cases of severe direct trauma (for example, with vertebral fracture), the different compressive mechanisms that will be mentioned later represent various aspects of a single degenerative phenomenon of the lumbar osteo-artro-discal complex. The nucleus pulposus is made up of a gelatinous material qualitatively similar - in terms of mucopolysaccharide content - to the cartilage of the vertebral plates from which it is nourished by imbibition. Nutrition is favoured by a periodic decompression mechanism connected to the spine's movements. The

---

[1] The yellow colour comes from the high content of elastin, which tends to decrease with age.

[2] The data is consistent with a well-known clinical finding: the "lumbar puncture" used for cerebro-spinal fluid withdrawals, injections of contrast media, or medications is painless.

nucleus is moderately acidic, with a pH of around 5.5, and is the largest avascular structure in the human body.

Note that the nucleus material is immunologically "segregated"; therefore, if it leaks out, it is identified as non-self and generates a significant inflammatory reaction. Occasionally, vessels can be found in persons under 20–30 years old. The nucleus can become vascularised in case of infectious processes (typically, a septic discitis, postoperative or from a remote infectious focus), thus becoming a source of intense pain. Cartilaginous ageing involves dehydration and reduction in the thickness of the nucleus. The annulus also weakens, becoming more extensible and less elastic with age, like any other ligament. The posterior joints collide due to the reduced spacing and begin to produce osteophytes.

The annulus does not have its algogenic innervation but is substantially fused with the posterior longitudinal ligament, which is provided instead. Laterally, it is in contact with the dural sheaths in the conjugation foramina. Consequently, disc alterations (protrusions or fissures) can be painful.

4.1.3 Protrusion or Disc Herniation

There are no clear criteria to differentiate a disc "protrusion" or "bulging" from a disc "herniation" unless the nucleus leaks out and the annuls (in which case, an "extruded" hernia is diagnosed). Disc protrusion (which from now on will also be defined as hernia for simplicity) can be a causal factor of much of the lumbar or "sciatic" pain, but this does not mean at all that every hernia is so. Most disc protrusions or hernias are entirely asymptomatic (or return asymptomatic after having caused problems). There seems to be a peak prevalence between 35 and 55 years old [3], so disc herniation is not a senile pathology. The herniation presupposes that the disc is still present and possibly moderately hydrated. At the same time, there must have already been a certain "wear" of the annulus and the posterior longitudinal ligament. This does not exclude that symptomatic disc hernias can also be found at very young and advanced ages, depending on the degree of disc dehydration.

The hernia's chronological sequence (entirely schematic) shows it begins to weaken the annulus and partially detach the adjacent posterior longitudinal ligament. The annulus can be torn ("fissured"), while usually the ligament, although partially detached from the annulus and - cranially or caudally - from the "posterior wall" of the vertebra, holds. If the ligament detaches sufficiently or is torn, a story of an extruded hernia can begin (not necessarily). The tension caused by the annulus and ligament can generate compressive pain. Suppose the pulpy nucleus leaks out of the annulus. In that case, there is also a pain of chemical and inflammatory origin justified (as already mentioned) by the acidity of the annulus itself and the immunogenicity of its content.

The compression can involve the dural sac, even if, fortunately, it rarely compresses the roots of the cauda significantly. Even the dural sac can become painful, especially if the chemical irritation reaches it directly or through an inflamed posterior longitudinal ligament.

The disc herniation can be median or lateralised to varying degrees. If it is median, it typically produces lower back pain. If the hernia lateralises, it can cause pain in the radicular or similar-radicular territory (always keep in mind the possibility that the pain is "referred" rather than frankly "radiating"). In extreme cases, the hernia can slip right into the conjugation foramen, already crowded by the presence of the spinal ganglion and roots, or even reach an "extra"-foraminal position in contact with what is now a spinal nerve generated by the confluence of the motor and post-ganglionic sensory fibres.

4.1.4   Why Hernias of the Fourth or Fifth Lumbar Disc Prevail

The posterior longitudinal ligament is a robust connective band that runs and adheres to all vertebrae's posterior face, ending at the lumbosacral junction. Thanks to its width, it practically covers the entire annulus up to about the L2 level. Caudally, it narrows, assuming a triangular frontal section ("tapering"). This anatomical peculiarity not only makes the ligament weaker in the caudal lumbar tracts, but, at the L4 and L5 levels, it practically leaves the lateral ends of the annulus uncovered. This explains why about 80% of disc herniations form at the fourth or fifth disc level. A herniation is more frequent at the fourth rather than at the fifth disc because the L4-L5 joint is more mobile.

4.1.5   Paralysing Sciatica

Hernias of the fourth or, less frequently, the fifth lumbar disc present a higher risk of complications with the so-called "paralysing (or paralytic) sciatica". The paralysis typically affects the leg muscles innervated by the L5 root. The patient suffers from sciatica and sometimes presents a modest deficit of dorsal flexion, particularly of the big toe. Suddenly, there is severe paresis of the extensor of the big toe, the common extensor of the fingers and the pedidius (the tibialis anterior may be less involved because an L4 radicular contingent innervates it). The phenomenon is presumably caused by a radicular infarct (the precariousness of the cauda's vascularisation will be discussed later). An axonal damage is generated, partly or entirely irreversible. For this reason, it is doubtful that the excision of the disc herniation can facilitate recovery once the paralysis has set in [5]. The surgical indication is there, but the operation must be performed urgently, ideally not beyond 72 h from the onset of paralysis [6]. I will discuss later how the doctor can behave in these risky cases.

4.1.6   Osteophytosis of the "facets" (Interapophyseal or Zygapophyseal Arthritis)

It has already been said that the reduction of disc thickness involves a progressive increase in the overlap between the articular facets, already subjected to considerable compressive and sliding stresses (their orientation favours the movements of flexion extension and partly of lateral lumbar flexion). Therefore, degeneration of the vertebral complex includes the enlargement of the facets due to osteophytic appositions, the thickening of the articular capsule and sometimes an intra-articular effusion that can even generate synovial cysts. If the cysts project towards the vertebral canal, these can compress the nerve roots as much or more than a protrusion.

The arthritis of the facets (or "interapophyseal" arthritis) can cause some pain in itself, but this is hardly a significant problem. The enlargement of the joints causes problems for its quota that reduces the section of the vertebral canal, thus determining the picture of a "narrow canal" or "stenosis", which has been discussed above: a pathological condition in which the motor deficit (spinal claudication) prevails and not the pain. Stenosis can be completely independent of a disc protrusion: disc dehydration, as mentioned, is already sufficient to cause excessive collision and overlap between the facets. Any protrusion further reduces the section of the vertebral canal. As already recalled, this form of arthritis generates, in CT or MRI images on the transverse plane (axial projections), a classic "triangle" shape of the spinal canal section (otherwise roughly round) as the osteophytes protrude inward. Even more typically, the canal takes on a "clover" shape because the conjugation holes are also reduced and transformed into narrow bony "channels" (Fig. 2.1).

This form of stenosis is called "acquired" because the canal is originally of normal size. Typically, the anteroposterior dimension remains normal or is slightly reduced, while the transverse section decreases significantly: the canal becomes more "narrow" than short. As mentioned, rare forms of congenital stenosis are caused by short pedicles (the bone passages between facets and the vertebral body). The situation is typical of achondroplasia, where severe and disabling stenosis can occur. However, stenosis of individual vertebrae can also be observed in non-achondroplastic subjects. The pedicles are the site of growth cartilage, and something can go wrong during development.

The "congenital" narrowed canal has a reduced anteroposterior diameter but generally maintains a more rounded shape (essentially, in axial projection, it appears shorter than narrower). It should be noted that the levels most exposed to acquired stenosis are L2-L3 and L3-L4, while the levels most exposed to disc herniation are L4-L5 and L5-S1. The reason is that the hinge axis for the flexion-extension of the lumbar spine is constituted by the joints between L2 and L3 and between L3 and L4, and this leads to a more intense effort on the respective inter apophyseal joints. The detail is relevant: if a CT study only extends between L3 and S1 (levels most suspected of disc herniation), one can miss the image of an overlying stenosis. As a rule, with MRI, the lumbar spine is taken entirely, but sometimes the images of cranial axial sections concerning L3 are not provided to the are not patient along with the report.

4.2 Muscle Pain

In low back pain and sciatica, the patient locates the pain in the lumbar muscle masses or lower limbs. In the case of the lower limbs, a skin or bone location can also be frequent. Often, especially at the paravertebral level, the muscles are actively contracted. In the case of low back pain, the spine images in X-ray or MRI often show (a detail not always reported) a noticeable flattening of the physiological lumbar lordosis (therefore, a de-lordotization). This is an automatic defensive (nocifensive) mechanism based on reducing intervertebral mobility.

Certainly, muscles contracted for a long time can generate pain of ischemic origin, but pain's "muscular" origin is absolutely overestimated. The pain is usually generated by the above-mentioned structures and placed inside the spinal canal. Therefore, it is only referred (or radiated) to neuromeric territories in the corresponding muscular or cutaneous metameres.

4.3 Meningeal Pain

The meningeal origin of pain is strongly underestimated. The lumbar dural sac (or dura mater) is innervated by the recurrent meningeal nerves of Luschka, as mentioned above. Like all visceral structures, the dural sac also refers to pain in territories far from the actual injury site. In this specific case, the uncertainty is increased by the capricious anatomy of the Luschka nerve.

The anatomy of the this nerve, first described in 1850 by Hubert von Luschka, still needs to be discovered, at least as far as the innervation of the dura mater [1, 7, 8] is concerned. Spinal nerves generate these "recurrent" nerves, which carry small-diameter unmyelinated sensory fibres (with a diameter around one or a few microns), both somatic and orthosympathetic. Following their course within the spinal canal is very difficult for anatomists. This tiny bundle of fibres certainly innervates the posterior longitudinal ligament.

The posterior and the epidural space, occupied by fat and a dense venous network to which I shall return, then branches inextricably onto the anterior portion of the dural sac, intersecting with the terminations of recurring nerves re-entering at multiple levels. In particular, the nerve that re-enters at level L2, and sometimes that of only one side, certainly bifurcates into an ascending and descending branch, practically covering the five lumbar levels. This explains the poor reliability of localising a disc herniation based on the site of reported pain or the Lasègue sign (which indeed "stretches" the dural sac while lengthening the sciatic nerve and its roots). Meningeal suffering originating at the lumbar level L2 can be attributed to dermatome L5 and vice versa.

The quality of the pain is reminiscent of visceral pains: poorly describable and associated with vegetative phenomena such as sweating and nausea. However, the defence mechanism reveals the meningeal origin of the pain. The dural sac is extensible, as is the entire spinal-radicular system. In the flexion of the lumbar spine, the system lengthens by several centimetres, and so must the dural sac, forcibly. If the dura is inflamed, any attempt to lengthen it generates intense pain (Chap. 2 discussed the Lasègue and Kernig signs as "meningeal" signs). This pain sends an alarm signal related to the central nervous system and prevails over any other form of pain. The patient will, therefore, try to keep the dural sac slackened. This goal can only be achieved with hyper-extension of the lumbar spine and, if necessary, of the cervical one.

Therefore, meningeal pain will produce the clinical phenotype that has been defined above as the "extensor patient." Conversely, an extensor phenotype strongly suggests a meningeal origin of the pain.

References

1. Bogduk N. The innervation of the lumbar spine. Spine. 1983;8(3):286–93.
2. Wyke B. The neurology of low back pain. In: The lumbar spine and back pain; Churchill Livingstone, UK: 1987. p. 265–339.
3. Frymoyer JW. Back pain and sciatica. N Engl J Med. 1988;31:291–300.
4. Mapp PI. Innervation of the synovium. Ann Rheum Dis. 1995;54:398–403.
5. Dubourg G, Rozenberg S, Fautrel B, Valls-Bellec I, Bissery A, Lang T, et al. A pilot study on the recovery from paresis after lumbar disc herniation. Spine. 2002;27(13):1426–31.
6. Yüksel MO, Çevik S. The effect of time elapsed from the onset of symptoms to surgery on prognosis in patients with foot drop due to lumbar disc Hernia. Duzce Med J. 2019;21(3):177–80.
7. Edgar MA, Nundy S. Innervation of the spinal dura mater. J Neurol Neurosurg Psychiatry. 1966;29(6):530–4.
8. Kaplan EB. Recurrent meningeal branch of the spinal nerves. Bull Hosp Jt Dis. 1947;8(1):108–9.

The Missing Link: Epidural Venous stasis $\qquad$ 5

5.1 Batson's Epidural Venous Plexus: Brief History and Anatomy

In 1940, the American surgeon Oscar V. Batson published a fundamental anatomical study that clearly described a fourth venous system present in the human body and in the Macacus rhesus monkey in addition to the caval, portal, and pulmonary systems [1].

There had been sporadic reports in the nineteenth century [2], but they were not systematic, especially not in vivo.

The first clear description of the epidural venous plexus is due to the French anatomist and surgeon Gilbert Breschet, a student of the famous Guillaume Dupuytren, Napoleon's doctor. Breschet described the plexus in a competitive essay in 1819 [3]. As suggested by some, it would perhaps be right to call this anatomical structure the Breschet-Batson plexus, even if until Batson, Breschet's discovery went unnoticed [2]. Isolated reports of "varicose" epidurals were not lacking subsequently, even if disconnected from Breschet's work. See, for example, an article by the American surgeon Charles A. Elsberg in 1916 [4], who cites the German anatomist Carl Samuel Wilhelm Gaup: Gaup in 1888 spoke of "haemorrhoids of the spinal dura mater" (I was not able to find Gaup's original work but the hemorrhoidal analogy is fitting indeed).

After Batson's publication, reports of "varicose" epidural veins have accumulated. For the 1950s, Pierre Wertheimer can be cited [5]. Some authors then classified epidural venous dilations into simple varices, thrombosed, and epidural hematoma [6]. In this text, several other examples will be cited. However, no neurosurgical case series have included "varicose" epidurals in the broader context of Batson's plexus anatomy: a context that opens up conservative therapeutic possibilities not limited to local surgery of the varices themselves. A recent review can be found in Hassan et al. [7].

© The Author(s), under exclusive license to Springer Nature Switzerland AG 2025

L. Tesio, *Low Back Pain and Sciatica*, https://doi.org/10.1007/978-3-031-78534-4_5

Batson was not interested in lower back pain but in the territorial distribution, somehow "paradoxical", of metastases of various forms of cancer. For example, metastases from prostate carcinoma often have initial vertebral or cranial theca locations and not - as one might expect - in the liver. With ingenious and accurate anatomical and contrastographic studies on human corpses and a single living monkey, he demonstrated that a long venous plexus connects the pelvis to the superior vena cava (therefore, to the right atrium) through the epidural space. This plexus is connected to the veins of the vertebral bodies, intracranial and intercostal, and therefore also to the azygos and the superior and inferior vena cava. The plexus has a reticular shape that reproduces the meshes of its structure at each vertebral level (Fig. 5.1), and, a significant detail, it is devoid of anatomical valves even if

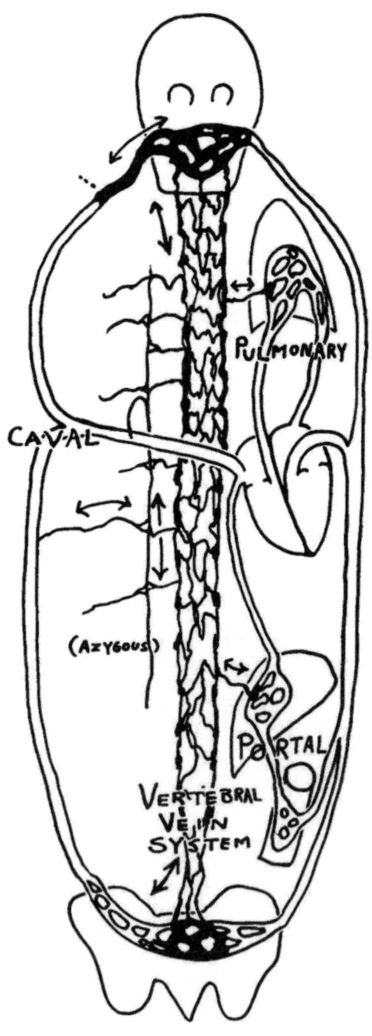

Fig. 5.1 The original figure of the article where Batson described the epidural venous plexus as the fourth venous system. From Batson, 1940 [1], with permission

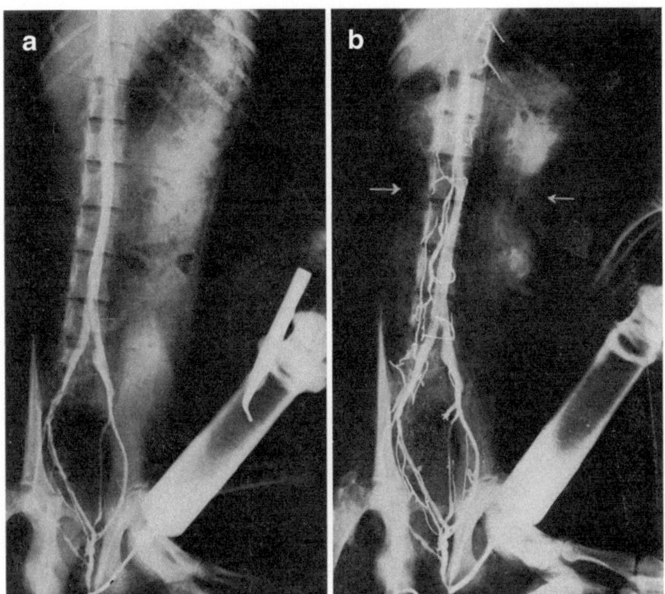

Fig. 5.2 Images from the article where Batson described the epidural venous plexus as the fourth venous system. The radiographic images show the distribution of contrast fluid injected in vivo into the dorsal vein of a monkey's penis (Macacus rhesus). On the left (**a**): baseline conditions. On the right (**b**): the abdominal pressure increases by tightening a towel around the animal's hips. In this latter case, a significant amount of venous blood is diverted towards the epidural venous plexus. From Batson, 1940 [1], with permission

"functional" valves (essentially appropriate angles) hinder craniocaudal filling, for example during efforts with the upper limbs.

Batson demonstrated that in the macaque, it was sufficient to slightly increase the abdominal pressure with a band to divert a considerable amount of venous blood towards the epidural plexus that would otherwise have preferably entered the caval system (Fig. 5.2). It was deduced that even simple Valsalva manoeuvres (a sneeze or a cough) could have the same effect in humans: to open the epidural route, virtually empty, to venous outflow. Surprisingly, an entire venous system could be the subject of a macro-anatomical discovery in the 1940s, but, as often happens, in reality, Batson arrived at least second after Breschet.

However, it took over 40 years before Batson's work received some attention from the scientific community. His anatomical findings were widely confirmed [8] through sophisticated cadaver studies (Figs. 5.3 and 5.4) that added interesting details. The plexus appears much more developed anteriorly than posteriorly. Moreover, its transverse veins run posterior to the posterior longitudinal ligament and close to the disc. They run between the ligament and the bone at the level of the posterior wall of the vertebral bodies.

A clear didactic scheme of the epidural venous plexus at the lumbar level (Fig. 5.5) can be found in a recent and well-documented review [9].

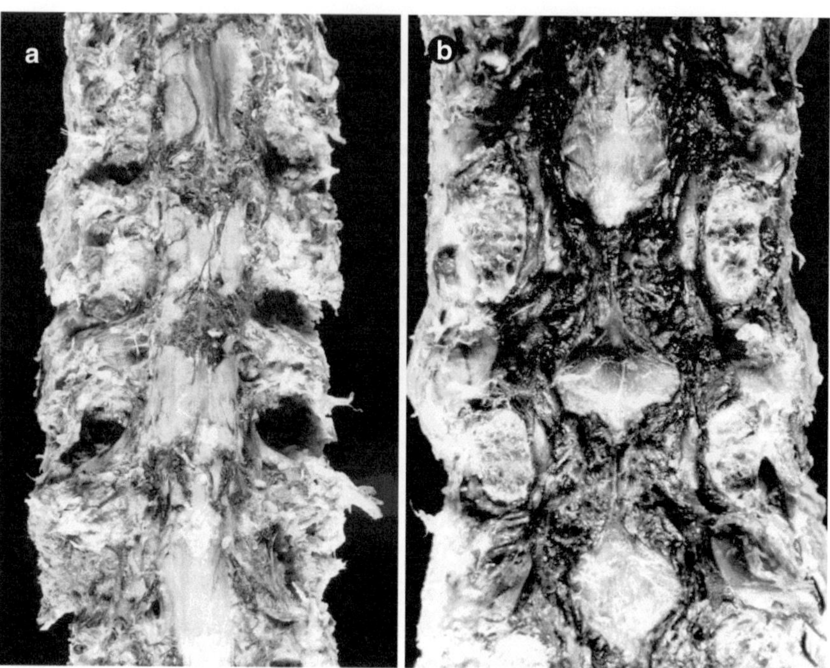

Fig. 5.3 Anatomical study on the epidural venous plexus (lumbar tract). On the left (**a**) posterior portion; on the right (**b**) anterior portion of the lumbar tract of the plexus. From Groen et al., 1997 [8], with permission

There have also been studies on humans in vivo. Before the era of MRI, venography was used to study disc protrusions that can "interrupt" some meshes of the epidural venous network. Today, it is possible (though, neglected in the literature) to study the venous plexus through an MRI or angio-MRI. The dilation of the venous plexus has been associated with various clinical conditions, some of which will be given in the following paragraphs. In all these conditions, lumbar or sciatic pain is almost a constant. In the following Chapters, particular attention will be paid to the role of epidural venous stasis in lumbosciatic pain: a role still very much underestimated.

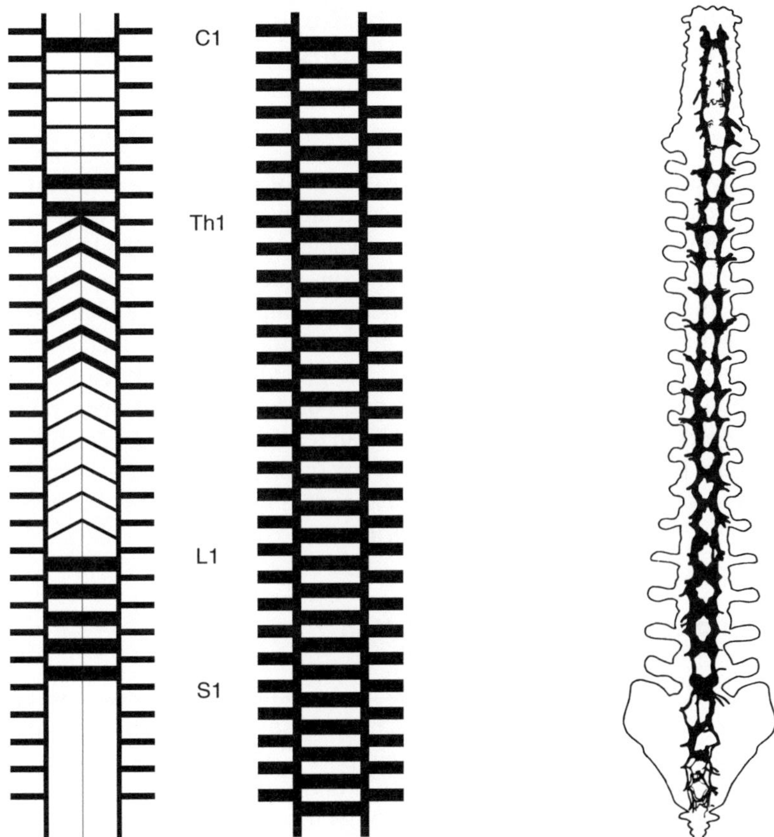

Fig. 5.4 Diagram of the distribution of the entire epidural venous plexus from the cervical to the sacral tract. On the left: the posterior portion of Batson's plexus; in the centre: the anterior portion; on the right: the schematic graphic reconstruction of the anterior portion of the plexus. From Groen et al., 1997 [8], with permission

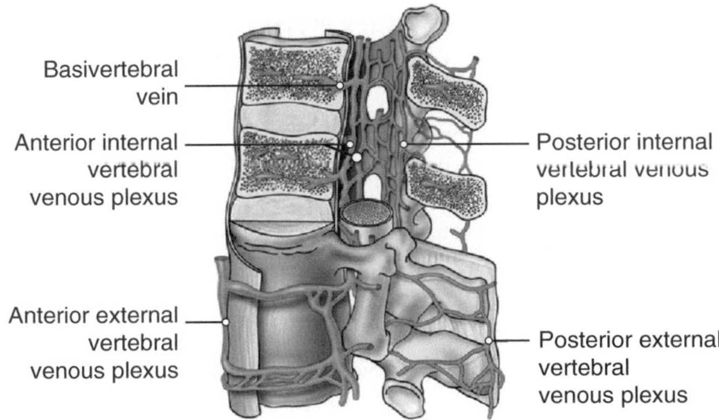

Fig. 5.5 Diagram of the epidural venous plexus at the lumbar level. From Carpenter et al., 2021 [9], with permission

5.2 Lumbar Pain and Dilation of the Epidural Venous Plexus: some Clinical Conditions

5.2.1 Pregnancy

From the twelfth week of pregnancy, about 50% of pregnant women suffer from lumbar or sciatic pain of varying duration and intensity, often persisting even after childbirth and very disabling [10]. Pregnant women do not have a higher prevalence of disc hernias than non-pregnant women: consequently, the explanation for this disorder remains controversial [11]. There is ample evidence that pregnancy involves dilation of the epidural venous plexus, both due to the increased venous flow directed towards the vena cava from the gravid uterus and due to the direct compression that the caval system undergoes. For decades, it has been known that in the last weeks, the caval venous pressure can reach, in the supine position, 20 cm H_2O (against the 4–5 cm H_2O in the absence of pregnancy) [12]. Therefore, the epidural venous plexus is an important escape route for the physiological excess of venous flow. The pain probably has this origin.

5.2.2 Inferior Vena Cava Obstruction

Thrombosis of the vena cava is known to cause significant dilations of the epidural venous plexus [13]. The prevalence of this mechanism has been estimated at around 1.3 per 1000 cases of lumbar or sciatic pain [14]. Considering the high prevalence of these syndromes, this is not an irrelevant proportion.

Figure 5.6 provides two examples. The MRI images show epidural venous dilation at the L5 level (sagittal and axial projection, A and B, respectively) at the top; in C, the resolution of the picture after unblocking of the vena cava is highlighted; in D (another patient), a noticeable dilation of the vena cava associated with intra-foraminal venous dilation at the lumbar level, is noted.

5.2.3 Heart Failure and Pulmonary Hypertension

The American physiatrist Myron LaBan is credited with the in-depth study of the association between venous stasis in internal conditions and lumbar pain. In exquisite publications, he highlighted the association between lumbosciatic pain and heart failure (and the rise of one of its biomarkers, the atrial natriuretic B-peptide) [15, 16], chronic obstructive pulmonary disease [17], nocturnal lumbar pain and also restless legs syndrome, which will be mentioned again later [16, 18, 19].

A cardiac deficit in "disposing" of venous return (right atrium in heart failure, right ventricle in pulmonary hypertension) causes an upstream venous stasis. The epidural venous plexus, it will be remembered, is a-valvular and therefore transmits as a "water hammer" any increase in central venous pressure (even that caused by a sneeze or a cough). The onset of lumbosciatic symptoms in all the clinical conditions mentioned above will depend, as a rule, on the concomitance of several

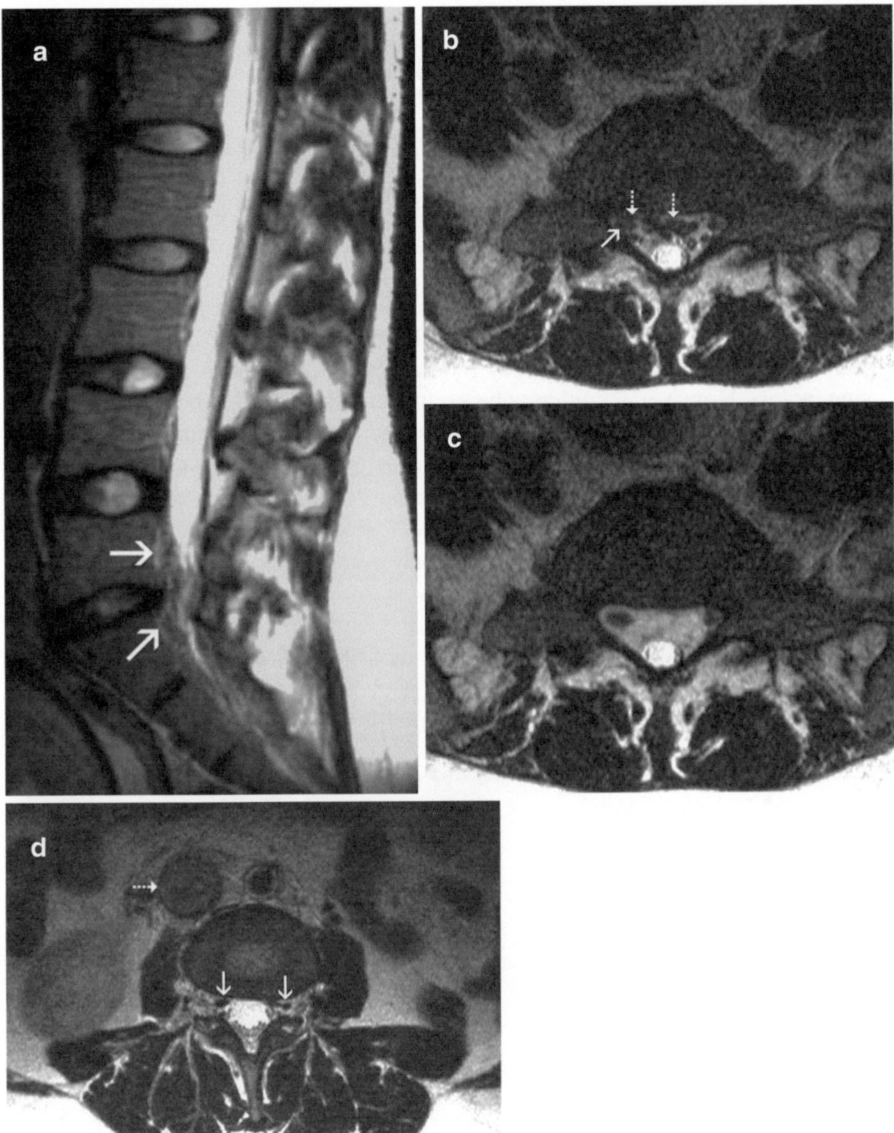

Fig. 5.6 MRI images of the epidural venous plexus dilation in two inferior vena cava obstruction cases. In the top left (**a**), the posterior displacement of the dural sac (white arrows) at level L5-S1 is noted; in the top right (**b**), the dilation of the epidural venous plexus (dashed white arrows) and the compression of the right S1 root (solid white arrow) is noted. In the bottom right (**c**), the venostasis resolution is noted after unblocking the inferior vena cava. In the bottom left (**d**) (another patient), dilation of the vena cava (dashed white arrow) associated with dilation of the radicular veins in the conjugation foramina (solid white arrows) is noted. From Paksoy and Gormus, 2004 [14], with permission

predisposing factors such as a narrow lumbar canal, otherwise asymptomatic disc protrusions or simply a prolonged decline position that in itself involves a higher epidural venous pressure than the one in an upright position. Rest removes a "muscle pump" effect, particularly paravertebral, and hinders further venous outflow.

5.3   The Venous Theory of "simple" Lumbar or Sciatic pain: An Unfinished Story

Epidural venous stasis, therefore, from the '80s of the last century, appears as a mediator between central venous stasis and lumbosciatic pain. These are, however, relatively rare situations because they require the concomitance of several predisposing factors. However, it could not be excluded that epidural venous stasis was the main causal factor, or co-causal with lumbar disc herniation, in the much more frequent forms of lumbosciatic pain without other extra-spinal clinical conditions. I explicitly stated this theory in 1991 [20], which was also proposed by LaBan in 1999 [19].

This idea opened up to an interpretation that went beyond the hydraulic pathogenetic mechanism, or venous stasis that causes compression and/or ischemia, also hypothesising a thrombophlebitic-inflammatory sequel to the stasis itself: from here stem some hints at therapeutic solutions that will be discussed later.

Figure 5.7, taken from a study by LaBan in 2001, shows venous angio-MRI images of the lumbar tract. This is a patient with left lumbosciatic pain refractory

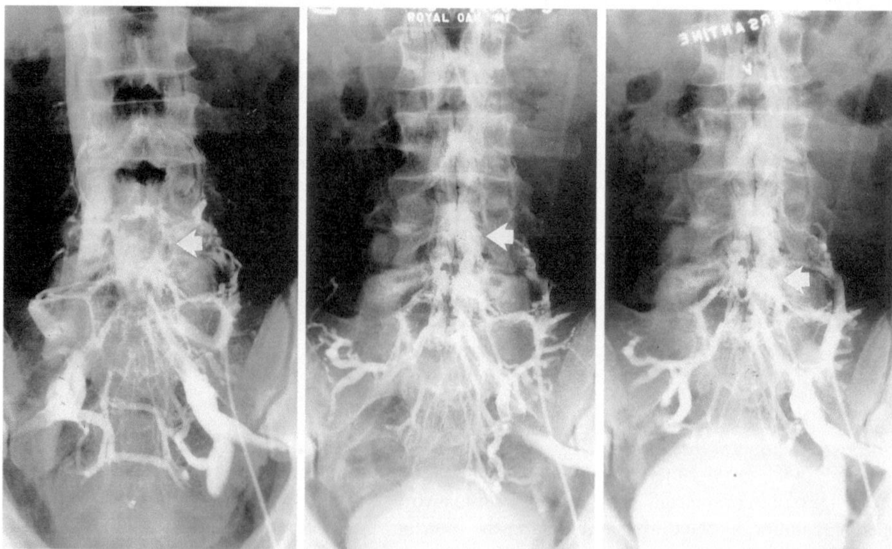

Fig. 5.7 Patient with left lumbosciatica refractory to various treatments for over 7 years, with all traditional tests negative (see text). Venous MRI angiography of the lumbar spine. On the left: marked dilation of the epidural venous plexus. In the centre, there is an increase in dilation with the Valsalva manoeuvre, associated with increased pain. On the right: further increase in dilation and pain with infusion of dipyridamole, a vasodilator. From LaBan et al., 2001 [21], with permission

("intractable") to the most various treatments for over 7 years. The instrumental exams were negative (CT, MRI, EMG, somatosensory evoked potentials, bone scintigraphy, pelvic ultrasound). The white arrows indicate the area of interest. On the left is an evident dilation of the Batson plexus at levels L4 and L5. In the centre, there is an increase in epidural vasodilation in response to a Valsalva manoeuvre that - coincidentally - exacerbates the pain. On the right, there is an even greater dilation, with even more intense pain, in response to the infusion of a vasodilator drug (dipyridamole). LaBan does not write about whether and how this patient finally found an effective therapy. To my knowledge, he has never proposed a therapeutic theory, consequent to the "venous" pathophysiological model, in his many studies. He concludes his article hoping for the end of the "unhealthy anatomical dogma of the 'tyranny of the herniated disc'".

The somewhat emotional conclusion of this article perhaps reflects the disappointment for the minimal (perhaps it would be better to say null) listening from the scientific community to this pathogenetic proposal. Yet the evidence has progressively accumulated but always in the form of individual cases or small series of cases, often focused on "varicose" epidural veins that generate pictures of lumbosacral radiculopathy similar to those generated by disc herniation [22–24]. New MRI techniques would now be able to highlight epidural venous stasis, particularly in the form of narrow canals [25, 26], but the idea is still foreign to clinical practice.

5.3.1   Narrow Lumbar Canal and Epidural Venous Stasis

It has already been reported that LaBan's studies [16] have focused attention on the possibility that the various symptoms of the syndrome from the narrow canal (spinal claudication, "restless legs," and, of course, low back pain) may depend on epidural venostasis. This more than reasonable hypothesis has been corroborated by an interesting in vivo study in which epidural pressure (level L5/S1) was measured during walking in subjects with a narrow lumbar canal or with a canal of normal dimensions [27].

Epidural pressure varies with the phases of the step and reaches a peak during the double support phase when, coincidentally, there is also maximum lumbar lordosis. In patients, the peak of epidural pressure was, on average, 250% higher than that of healthy subjects (83 versus 34 mmHg). Walking in a slightly flexed position (preferred by patients), subjects with a narrow canal achieved a marked drop in epidural pressure. The pressure reached that of the control subjects in upright trunk walking. Even in healthy subjects, walking in flexion produced a drop in the peak epidural pressure, but to a modest extent (from 34 to 27 mmHg). These are pressures that, albeit intermittently, are still sufficient to occlude local venous circulation.

This data provides a pathophysiological basis for widespread observations. For example, patients with low back pain often report attenuation or disappearance of pain if they exert themselves with a flexed trunk, such as walking uphill, cycling, or pushing heavy carts. Conversely, they report that pain appears or intensifies for much lesser efforts but is performed upright or extended (for example, walking downhill). This dependence on the more or less extended position of the lumbar spine is widespread in cases of disc protrusion and is almost the rule in cases of a narrow lumbar canal.

5.3.2   An Interesting Corollary: Cervical Pain and Headache

LaBan has highlighted how epidural venous stasis can generate problems even at the cervical level [25]. Even the epidural venous stasis seems to mediate the headache that, quite mysteriously, can be associated with the compression of the left renal vein in the "nutcracker" constituted by the angle between the aorta and the superior mesenteric artery (the "nutcracker syndrome").

The mystery clears up, once again, if we consider the epidural venous plexus. Unlike the right renal vein, the left renal vein receives several tributary veins that "discharge" through it: for example, the gonadal veins (the syndrome should be suspected in case of varicocele associated with left side pain and intermittent micro/macrohematuria). Here, veins communicating with the second lumbar vein should be mentioned. And again, the third lumbar vein is often grafted right onto the renal vein. An obstacle to renal outflow can, therefore, generate a "leak" of venous blood towards the Batson plexus up to generate its dilation sub-occipital and at the cranial base (hence the headache, typically in the supine position when the cervical and cephalic venous pressure increase) [28].

5.3.3   A Suspicious Association: Low Back Pain and Erectile Dysfunction Therapy

In recent years, the use of phosphodiesterase inhibitors for the treatment of erectile dysfunction has spread. Essentially, these drugs cause sustained penile veno-dilation. Their selectivity, however, is not total. Side effects related to systemic vasodilation are known: typically nasal congestion. Among the side effects is the onset of low back pain (incidence between 3% and 9%). Although transient, this complication is still among the first 20 side effects described in the first month of treatment and among the first 20 causes of treatment abandonment with tadalafil [29, 30].

The mechanism by which these drugs cause low back pain is described as "unknown," but it is straightforward to recognise an epidural veno-dilation in it. Incidentally, it is reasonable to expect that the incidence of the complication is much higher in cases of a narrow lumbar canal (indeed, the therapy could even reveal clinically latent stenosis). Still, I have not found specific evidence in the literature.

5.3.4   Evidence of Critical Circulation in the Ganglia and Roots of the Cauda

Interesting anatomical studies have shown how ensuring venous return is also fundamental at the level of the roots of the cauda.

Recalling the anatomical peculiarity of the vascularisation of roots and ganglia is appropriate. The spinal roots (not the ganglia) present a blood-nerve barrier similar to the blood-brain one. If these are intact, histological protein tracers and contrast media for MRI penetrate the ganglia but not into the roots. However, an external compression that generates venous stasis "forces" the barrier and generates protein extravasation, and therefore, oedema can evolve into fibrosis [31].

Is it easy to obtain sufficient venous pressure? Yes, it is easy not only thanks to the rigid and restricted space in which the roots are located and, during the movements of the spine or lower limbs, flow (see also the already mentioned study on epidural pressure in walking) [27], but also thanks to the peculiar, very superficial distribution of the veins in the roots and the ganglia. Here, the arteries run mainly deep in the root and the ganglion, while the veins run on the periphery, which is the case in the central nervous system. In most other anatomical structures of the human body, arteries and veins are arranged in parallel in depth.

Another risk associated with venous compression is ischemia of arterial origin. It is curious how we talk about "cauda equina" relative to an anatomical structure (the lumbosacral roots) that has unique characteristics for the human species. It is specific to man, in fact, the relative shortening of the spinal cord compared to the spine during growth, a phenomenon that imposes a considerable length on the lumbosacral roots.

The roots of the cauda are subjected to lengthening and shortening of several centimetres during the daily movements of flexion and extension of the lumbar spine and pelvis. Therefore, one should ask how they manage to maintain their vascularisation, which is already quite precarious. The arterial flow comes from vessels of modest size, both from the radicular and anterior spinal arteries. Hence, the cauda roots' intermediate tract is a "watershed" territory at risk of ischemia [32, 33].

Parke and collaborators have shown that the lumbar roots are equipped with a particular artery-venous anastomotic system (Figs. 5.8 and 5.9) [34–36]. These spiral vessels ("pigtails") withstand stretching very well. If the arterial flow decreases, the problem can be solved by arterializing the vein downstream of the obstruction. This mechanism, however, requires that venous pressure is not so high as to prevent arterial flow in the new venous bed towards the periphery. Therefore, central, epidural and also peri-radicular venous stasis can generate ischemic damage on the roots (mechanism from which pain and neurological symptoms and signs derive) with a fourfold mechanism: direct compressive, compressive through perineural oedema, venous ischemia, arterial ischemia.

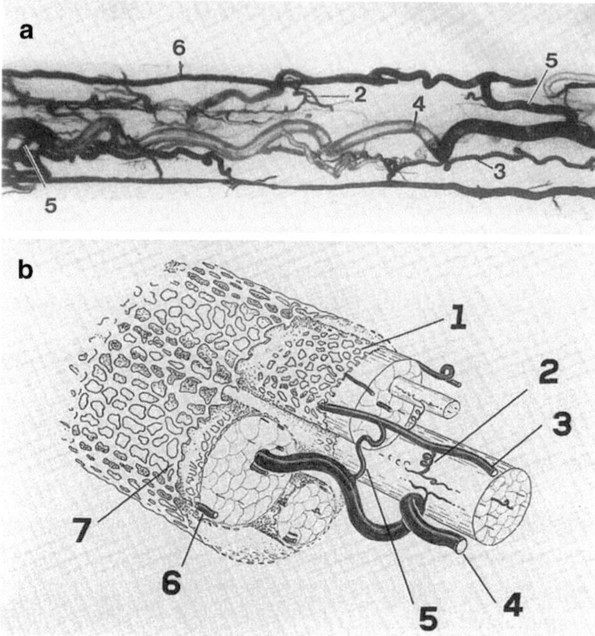

Fig. 5.8 Anatomy of the vascularisation of the lumbosacral roots. At the top is the microvascular study of a fourth lumbar root (dark arteries, light veins). Numerous arteriovenous anastomoses are noticeable. Below is a graphic diagram of the radicular anatomy inspired by Parke (2005) [36]. The characteristic spiral aspect of the anastomoses is highlighted, which are therefore able to adapt to the elongation of the roots during the flexion movements of the lumbar spine and the pelvis that involve the elongation of the sciatic nerve. 1, 7: pia-arachnoid; 2, 3, 6: arteries; 4: veins; 5: arteriovenous anastomoses. From Parke, 2005 [36], with permission

5.3.5 From Stasis to Phlebitis to Fibrosis, We Broaden the Field of Observation

At this point, perhaps there is more than enough evidence to favour epidural venous circulation's leading role in the low back and sciatic pain genesis. Yet this evidence continues not to arouse particular interest in the medical community. I will now try to add other evidence related to the inflammatory consequences of venostasis that most authors have not considered so far, despite their importance to venous stasis as the cause of compression and ischemia of allogenic terminations.

As is known, venous stasis is a decisive risk factor for phlebitic evolution, a common condition in the lower limbs and the hemorrhoidal plexus. It is well known that the process initially has an inflammatory nature, which then sees the deposition of fibrinogen and then fibrin. Fibrinolytic processes contrast this process, but venous stasis significantly breaks this constant dynamic balance if factors hinder fibrinolysis. These are the same factors (for example, sedentary lifestyle and smoking) that increase the risk of arterial thrombosis in coronary heart disease or stroke. These

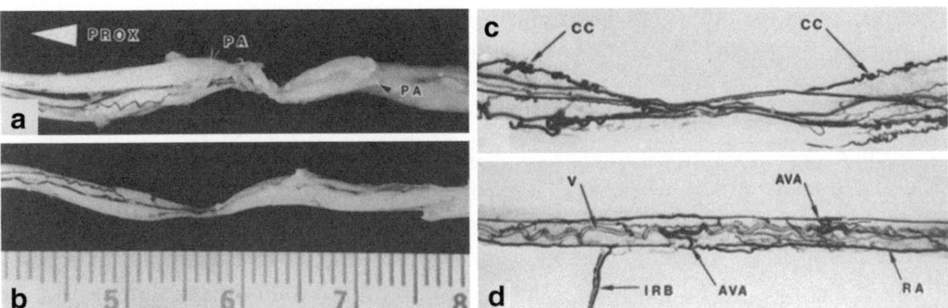

Fig. 5.9 The L5 and S1 radicular vascular system in a case of root compression. In (**a** and **b**): preparation in optical microscopy. In (**a**), the sensory and motor L5 roots adhered to each other at the compression site (with hypertrophy of the pia mater and arachnoid) are highlighted. In (**b**, the sensory root has been isolated: at the compression site, its thickness is reduced to 25% of the original (scale in cm). In (**c** and **d**): electron microscopy, S1 sensory root. In (**c**), surprisingly, the radicular arteries maintain their continuity. "Curls" (CC: compensating coils) are noticeable in the proximal and distal sections relative to the noticeable compression. Presumably, these spirals maintain the extensibility of the arteries themselves since the radicular elongation must be borne by the supra- and sublesional areas, given that the compressed area is fibrous and less extensible. In (**d**), the preparation produces dilation of the veins (recognisable because they are lighter). Large spiral arteriovenous anastomoses are noticeable, allowing blood passage from arteries to radicular veins. *PROX* proximal, *PA* pia-arachnoid, *V* veins, *AVA* arteriovenous anastomoses, *IRB* interradicular branches, *RA* radicular arteries. From Watanabe and Parke, 1986 [34], with permission

factors can result in a complete thrombosis of the dilated veins and a fibrotic connective evolution of the surrounding tissue.

The "leather-like" skin and subcutaneous tissue that results after severe phlebitis in the lower limbs is frequently encountered and easily observed. There is no reason to exclude that the epidural fat can evolve similarly if phlebitis (from stasis or inflammation caused by disc material) affects the epidural veins. This hypothesis was developed between the '80s and '90s of the last century by a group of English rheumatologists led by Malcolm V. Jayson.

It should be said immediately that, even in an era that already saw the spread of computers, network databases and emails, the "biochemical-inflammatory" line of thought and the "hydraulic-mechanical" line of thought never crossed their paths.

Jayson and his group demonstrated that:

- chronic low back pain is significantly associated with fibrinolytic deficit [37–40];
- the fibrotic tissue in cases of chronic low back pain, and even more after ineffective (or detrimental) surgical interventions, shows phlebitic and post-phlebitic alterations identical to those found in the subcutaneous post-phlebitic tissue of the lower limbs [39];
- in proof of the fact that disc pathology in chronic low back pain is associated with inflammatory phenomena, in the nucleus pulposus of many patients blood vessels and free nerve endings can be found that are absent in intact discs [41];

Therefore, the nucleus can become a source of pain in these particular cases.

In a single article, Jayson linked epidural venostasis and thrombophlebitic phenomena: a study on surgically removed discs [42]. Only in a brief Letter was venous dilation mentioned collaterally as a possible cause of low back pain [43]. Venostasis, in essence, was interpreted mainly as secondary and not as primitive compared to phlebitic/fibrotic phenomena. The hypothesised primary cause was a leakage of inflammatory molecules from inside a damaged disc [44].

The point of view was, therefore, purely biochemical. For example, in several works of Jayson's group, there is a certain ambiguity in defining "arachnoiditis" as the inflammatory processes of tissue samples taken post-mortem in patients who had suffered from chronic low back pain or of tissue samples removed during herniectomy. Arachnoiditis is a form of chronic meningitis that at the lumbar level incarcerates the roots of the cauda and is a very feared complication of surgical interventions or, rarely, of cerebrospinal fluid withdrawals. As already mentioned, at the time, arachnoiditis could also not be an exceptional consequence of myelographic studies with liposoluble contrast medium before water-soluble contrast media became available. In many cases, it is evident that the studied tissue could also be epidural fat.

No studies on therapeutic attempts based on pro-fibrinolytic drugs have been published. Towards the end of the '90s, this line of research ran out.

References

1. Batson OV. The function of the vertebral veins and their role in the spread of metastases. Ann Surg. 1940;112(1):138–49.
2. Nathoo N, Caris EC, Wiener JA, Mendel E. History of the vertebral venous plexus and the significant contributions of Breschet and Batson. Neurosurgery. 2011;69(5):1007–14.
3. Breschet G. Essay on the veins of the spine. Paris: Mequignon-Marvis; 1819.
4. Elsberg CA. The surgical significance and operative treatment of enlarged and varicose veins of the spinal cord. Am J Neurosurg. 1916;151:642–52.
5. Wertheimer P, Ravault P, Vignon G, Michel P. Sciatica and dilation of the epidural veins. Rev Rheum Osteoartic Dis. 1953;20(11):764–73.
6. Genevay S, Palazzo E, Huten D, Fossati P, Meyer O. Lumboradiculalgia due to epidural varices. About two cases. Review of the literature. Rev Rheumatol. 2002;69:308–12.
7. Hassan O, Lewis CS, Aradhyula L, Hirshman BR, Pham MH. Engorged venous plexus mimicking adjacent segment disease: case report and literature review. Surg Neurol Int. 2020;9(11):104.
8. Groen RJM, Groenewegen HJ, Van Alphen HAM, Hoogland PVJM. Morphology of the human internal vertebral venous plexus: a cadaver study after intravenous Araldite CY 221 injection. Anat Rec. 1997;249(2):285–94.
9. Carpenter K, Decater T, Iwanaga J, Maulucci CM, Bui CJ, Dumont AS, et al. Revisiting the vertebral venous plexus–A comprehensive review of the literature. World Neurosurg. 2021;145:381–95.
10. Ostgaard HC, Andersson GBJ, Karlsson K. Prevalence of back pain in pregnancy. Spine. 1991;16(5):549–52.
11. Weinreb JC, Wolbarsht LB, Cohen JM, Brown CE, Maravilla KR. Prevalence of lumbosacral intervertebral disk abnormalities on MR images in pregnant and asymptomatic nonpregnant women. Radiology. 1989;170(1 Pt 1):125–8.

12. Kerr M, Scott D, Samuel E. Studies of the inferior vena cava in late pregnancy. BMJ. 1964;1:532–3.
13. Bozkurt G, Cil B, Akbay A, Turk CC, Palaoglu S. Intractable radicular and low back pain secondary to inferior vena cava stenosis associated with Budd-Chiari syndrome: endovascular treatment with cava stenting: case report and review of the literature. Spine. 2006;31(12):E383–6.
14. Paksoy Y, Gormus N. Epidural venous plexus enlargements presenting with radiculopathy and back pain in patients with inferior vena cava obstruction or occlusion. Spine. 2004;29(21):2419–24.
15. LaBan MM, McNeary L. The clinical value of B-type natriuretic peptide (BNP) in predicting nocturnal low back pain in patients with concurrent lumbar spinal stenosis and cardiopulmonary dysfunction (Vesper's Curse): a clinical case series. Am J Phys Med Rehabil. 2008;87(10):798–802.
16. LaBan MM, Viola SL, Femminineo AF, Taylor RS. Restless legs syndrome associated with diminished cardiopulmonary compliance and lumbar spinal stenosis - a motor concomitant of "Vesper's curse". Arch Phys Med Rehabil. 1990;71(6):384–8.
17. LaBan MM, Kucway EJ. Aeolus myth: chronic obstructive lung disease and nocturnal lumbosacral pain in association with lumbar spinal stenosis and pulmonary hypertension. Am J Phys Med Rehabil. 2003;82(9):660–4.
18. LaBan M. "Vespers curse" night pain. The bane of Hypnos. Arch Phys Med Rehabil. 1984;65:501–4.
19. LaBan MM, Wang AM, Shetty A, Sessa GR, Taylor RS. Varicosities of the paravertebral plexus of veins associated with nocturnal spinal pain as imaged by magnetic resonance venography: a brief report. Am J Phys Med Rehabil. 1999;78(1):72–6.
20. Tesio L. The cause of back pain and sciatica can also be venous. Br J Rheumatol. 1991;XXX(1):70–1.
21. LaBan MM, Wilkins JC, Wesolowski DP, Bergeon B, Szappanyos BJ. Distention of the paravertebral venous plexus (Batson's): a causative agent in lumbar radiculopathy as observed by venous angiography. Am J Phys Med Rehabil. 2001;80(2):129–33.
22. Pennekamp M, Kraft CN, von Engelhardt LV, Lüring C, Schmitz APHG. Epidural varicose veins are a rare cause of acute radicular lumbar syndrome with complete foot drop and flexor paresis—case report and literature review. Z Orthop Unfall. 2007;145(01):55–60.
23. Qiang Z, Wenxue J. Epidural venous enlargements presenting with lumboradiculopathy. Joint Bone Spine. 2012;79:416–7.
24. Bursalı A, Akyoldas G, Guvenal AB, Yaman O. Lumbar epidural varix mimicking disc herniation. J Korean Neurosurg Soc. 2016;59(4):410–3.
25. LaBan MM, Wang AM. Engorgement of the cervical spinal epidural venous plexus simulating a spinal epidural mass. Am J Phys Med Rehabil. 2014;93(7):634–5.
26. Kamogawa J, Kato O, Morizane T. Three-dimensional visualization of internal vertebral venous plexuses relative to dural sac and spinal nerve root of spinal canal stenosis using MRI. Jpn J Radiol 2018; 36(5):351–360.
27. Takahashi K, Kagechica K, Takino T, Matsui T, Miyazaki T, Shima I. Changes in epidural pressure during walking in patients with lumbar spinal stenosis. Spine. 1995;20(24):2746–9.
28. Rozen TD, Devcic Z, Toskich B, Caserta MP, Sandhu SJS, Huynh T, et al. Nutcracker phenomenon with a daily persistent headache as the primary symptom: case series and a proposed pathogenesis model based on a novel MRI technique to evaluate for spinal epidural venous congestion. J Neurol Sci. 2022;434:120170.
29. Seftel A, Farber J, Fletcher J, Deeley MC, Elion-Mboussa A, Hoover A, et al. A three-part study to investigate the incidence and potential etiologies of tadalafil-associated back pain or myalgia. Int J Impot Res. 2005;17(5):455–61.
30. Hazell L, Cornelius V, Wilton LV, Shakir SAW. The safety profile of tadalafil as prescribed in general practice in England: results from a prescription-event monitoring study involving 16 129 patients. BJU Int. 2009;103(4):506–14.
31. Kobayashi S, Yoshizawa H, Hachiya Y, Ukai T, Morita T. Vasogenic edema induced by compression injury to the spinal nerve root. Spine. 1993;18(11):1410–24.

32. Parke WW, Gammell K, Rothman RH. Arterial vascularisation of the cauda equina. J Bone Joint Surg. 1981;63-A(1):53–62.
33. Namba K. Vascular anatomy of the cauda equina and its implication on the vascular lesions in the caudal spinal structure. Neurologia Medico-Chirurgica. 2016;56:310–6.
34. Watanabe R, Parke WW. Vascular and neural pathology of lumbosacral spinal stenosis. J Neurosurg. 1986;64:64–70.
35. Parke WW. The intrinsic vasculature of the lumbosacral spinal nerve roots. Spine. 1985;10(6):508–15.
36. Parke WW. Role of epidural and radicular veins in chronic back pain and radiculopathy. In: Kambin P, editor. Arthroscopic and endoscopic spinal surgery: text and atlas. 2nd ed. Totowa, NJ: Humana Press; 2005. p. 151–65.
37. Hoyland JA, Freemont AJ, Jayson MI. Intervertebral foramen venous obstruction. A cause of periradicular fibrosis. Spine. 1989;14(6):558–68.
38. Klimiuk PS, Pountain GD, Keegan AL, Jayson MI. Serial measurements of fibrinolytic activity in acute low back pain and sciatica. Spine. 1987;12(9):925–8.
39. Pountain GD, Keegan AL, Jayson MI. Impaired fibrinolytic activity in defined chronic back pain syndromes. Spine. 1987;12(2):83–6.
40. Jayson MI, Million R, Keegan A, Tomlinson I. A fibrinolytic defect in chronic back pain syndromes. Lancet. 1984;13:1186–7.
41. Freemont AJ, Peacock TE, Goupille P, Hoyland JA, O'Brien J, Jayson MI. Nerve ingrowth into diseased intervertebral disc in chronic back pain. Lancet. 1997;350(9072):178–81.
42. Cooper RG, Freemont AJ, Hoyland JA, Jenkins JP, West CG, Illingworth KJ, et al. Herniated intervertebral disc-associated periradicular fibrosis and vascular abnormalities occur without inflammatory cell infiltration. Spine. 1995;20(5):591–8.
43. Jayson MI. Mechanisms underlying chronic back pain. BMJ. 1994;309:681–2.
44. Goupille P, Jayson MI, Valat JP, Freemont AJ. The role of inflammation in disk herniation-associated radiculopathy. Semin Arthritis Rheum. 1998;28(1):60–71.

Part III

Explaining the Contradictions

Explaining the (Few) Different Clinical Pictures

6

6.1 Disc Mechanics

6.1.1 Disc Pressure: The Nucleus Pulposus Does Not Tell the Whole Story

The lumbar disc supports very high loads, as cadaver and in vivo studies demonstrated. In these latter studies, a pressure probe was inserted into the third lumbar disc of healthy volunteers. The pioneering works of Nachemson [1] have been replicated, and their results have been updated [2, 3]. Today, it can be considered that, in an adult weighing 65–75 kg, on the third or fourth lumbar disc in a sitting position, there is a load of 10 to 15 kg/cm^2 (currently, pressure is measured with the less popular Pascal: 1 Mega Pascal (MPa) is equivalent to 10.2 kg/cm^2). The pressure drops by 30% in static and 50% in supine position. The intradiscal pressure can rise to over 23 kg/cm^2 when lifting an object weighing 20 kg with a flexed trunk.

If one hypothesises a surface of the vertebral plate of 7–8 cm^2, it is immediately seen how the disc load exceeds one hundred kilograms in many acts of daily life. Note that cases of vertebral fractures are more frequent than cases of traumatic disc herniations (especially if osteopenia is present). On anatomical preparations, it is shown that on a healthy lumbar disc, the compressive force must exceed 500 kg before initial fissures are observed. Still, at that point, fractures have already occurred on the adjacent cartilaginous plates [4]. Therefore, if one wants to consider the disc among the direct or predisposing causes of low back pain, it is advisable to look at the degeneration of the annulus, which is entrusted with the containment of the nucleus, and to look at its mechanics, as will be motivated below.

© The Author(s), under exclusive license to Springer Nature Switzerland AG 2025
L. Tesio, *Low Back Pain and Sciatica*,
https://doi.org/10.1007/978-3-031-78534-4_6

6.1.2 The Mechanics of the Disc in Relation to Spine Movements

Understanding the mechanics of the disc in relation to spine movements is crucial. It provides a deeper insight into the biomechanics of the lumbar disc and its implications for low back pain.

It must always be remembered that the disc comprises the nucleus pulposus and the annulus fibrosus. The nucleus is not an incompressible liquid but a viscoelastic material whose hydration occurs through the cartilaginous plates and varies throughout the day. The nucleus is more hydrated upon waking, so an adult's height may be a couple of centimetres greater than that observed at night. What happens to the disc with movements of the lumbar spine? The most studied movements are those of flexion, extension and lateral flexion. The results for many years have been controversial also due to experimental difficulties and the diversity of methods adopted. Since their appearance, these studies on the "migration" of the nucleus have been the basis of exercise methods that have made it their rationale [5]: a (thorny) point to which we will return later.

Biomechanical studies have been conducted on anatomical samples, engineering models, and volunteers, both healthy and with sciatica, with different sample sizes (from single cases to hundreds of subjects). The studies on humans investigated various positions (sitting, supine, prone, erect) in static situations or during movements. The first in vivo studies used invasive discography (injection of contrast fluid into the disc), CT, and MRI. Soon, the prominent bone of contention became the direction of nucleus displacement during flexion or extension of the lumbar spine, according to the hypothesis that the displacement of the nucleus could be the basis of a subsequent herniation. For the interested reader and correctness, a brief list of articles supporting the contrasting versions is proposed in the bibliography [6–11]. On discs with various degrees of degeneration, protrusions of the annulus of 2–5 mm are described (Fig. 6.1 and Table 6.1) [12].

When studying the lumbar spine, it's essential to focus on the annulus rather than the nucleus. This is a key aspect in understanding disc protrusion and its implications for low back pain.

When studying the lumbar spine with an MRI of various positions of the trunk (flexion, extension, sitting or standing position), it is referred to as "dynamic" or kinetic MRI, kMRI [13, 14]. Thanks to these studies, in summary, it can be confirmed that disc protrusion occurs towards the concavity [12, 15]. Therefore, at least in discs that are not perfectly intact, in extension, the migration facilitates the posterior protrusion of the annulus (Fig. 6.2), which could eventually generate a clinically relevant protrusion. This understanding of the annulus's role in disc protrusion is crucial in our quest to comprehend and manage low back pain.

It should be reiterated that the role of the nucleus may still be secondary in generating disc protrusion compared to the role of the annulus, which is in line with anatomical studies that confirm a significant protrusion of the annulus itself in extension. To this, it must be added that the yellow ligaments also "sag" in extension, thus contributing to reducing the vertebral canal section (see further on).

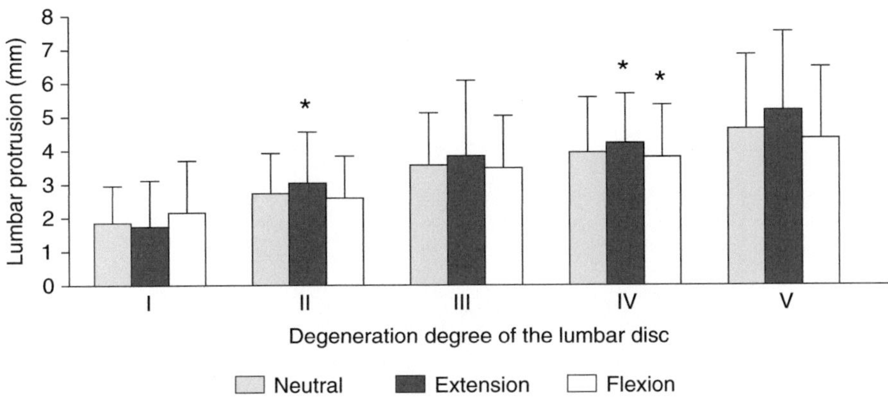

Fig. 6.1 Disc protrusion with flexion and extension of the lumbar spine. The study used a "dynamic" MRI, allowing trunk flexion-extension. L4/L5 segment. The results refer to 513 subjects with low back pain and/or sciatica. The histograms report the average disc protrusion relative to the posterior vertebral margin. The trunk was still under load. The degree of flexion or extension is not specified. In white: "neutral" upright position. In light grey: trunk flexion. In dark grey: extension. The asterisk indicates a significant difference compared to the "neutral" position. The ordinate reports the amplitude of the protrusion in millimetres without specifying its direction. The text specifies that only in discs with very initial signs of suffering (severity 1, see Table 6.1) does extension generate anterior protrusion, flexion posterior protrusion. In all other pathological conditions (gravity 2–5), flexion does not generate appreciable protrusions, while extension causes posterior disc protrusions (significant for conditions 2 and 4). The results are comparable to those of the other lumbar segments (not illustrated). Note that, in any case, the increase in posterior protrusion associated with the flexed position (present only in healthy discs: condition 1, dark grey bar), compared to the protrusion observable in the upright position, on average is less than one millimetre. From Zou et al., 2009, [12], with permission

Table 6.1 Classification of lumbar disc degeneration

Severity	Nucleus signal intensity	Nucleus structure	Distinction of nucleus and annulus	Disc height
1	Hyperintense	Homogeneous, white	Clear	Normal
2	Hyperintense	Heterogeneous with horizontal band, white	Clear	Normal
3	Intermediate	Heterogeneous, from grey to black	Not very clear	From normal to decreased
4	Hypointense	Heterogeneous, from grey to black	Lost	From normal to diminished
5	Hypointense	Heterogeneous, from grey to black	Lost	Collapsed

The table reports the classification criteria adopted by the authors to define the degrees of disc degeneration based on MRI findings, as on the x-axis of Fig. 6.1 (modified from Zou et al. 2009) [12]

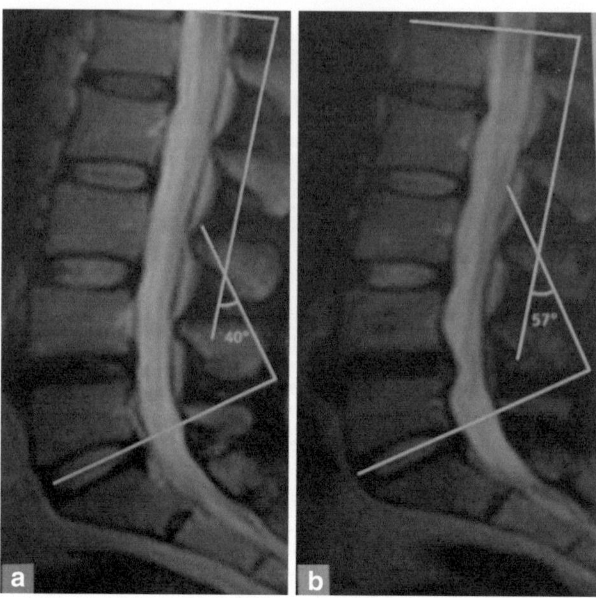

Fig. 6.2 Dynamic lumbo-sacral MRI (under load). Sagittal image of the lumbar spine in an asymptomatic subject but with initial L4/L5 disc degeneration (note the "black" disc; therefore, it is not as hydrated as the adjacent discs). On the left (**a**): "neutral" supine position. On the right (**b**): upright position. Due to the more significant lordosis, the dural sac takes on an anterior "scalloped" appearance created by the modest disc protrusions. There is also a frank protrusion at the L4/L5 disc level. From Michelini et al., 2018 [15], with permission

Understanding the migration of the nucleus during lateral flexion is crucial. It's a controversial yet significant aspect in disc protrusion and its implications for low back pain.

Torsion alone does not generate migration but generates tensile stress on the annulus, making it more prone to subsequent herniations. These conclusions largely confirm Brown's already mentioned engineering study on anatomical preparations, which is far in time but still fundamental [4]. In this study, some anatomical preparations of healthy lumbar segments were subjected to classic material resistance tests through various pressures and torsional tensions, flexo-extension, and lateral flexion. The authors demonstrated that the migration of the nucleus goes towards the concavity of the spine but, above all, formalised an even more important conclusion. The protrusion observed is due more to direct compression of the annulus from the concave side by the adjacent vertebral margins than to the "push" determined by the nucleus. This result was confirmed 31 years later by another crucial anatomical-biomechanical study (Fig. 6.3) [16].

Another much more recent in vivo study [17] confirmed the secondary role of the nucleus in disc deformations during spine movements. In a healthy lumbar disc, during movements of the lumbar spine, there is not an actual "migration" but only a deformation (a flattening-lengthening) of the nucleus, mainly forward, without

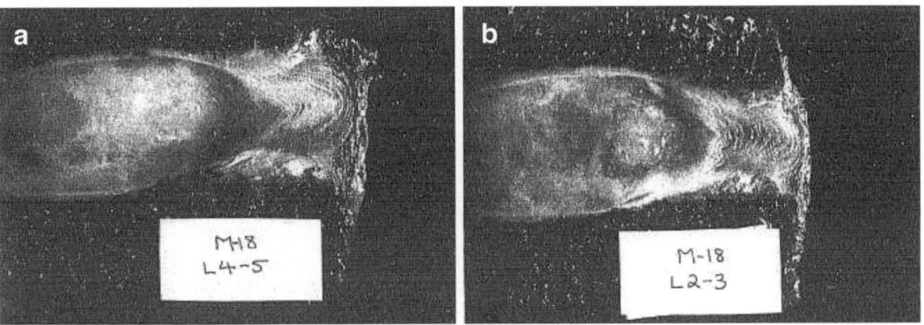

Fig. 6.3 Dynamic study on a corpse: effect on the lumbar spine's disc of extension and flexion. On the left (**a**): anatomical preparation of a sagittal section of the L4/L5 lumbar disc, in extension. On the right (**b**): sagittal section of the L2/L3 lumbar disc, in flexion. Note how the extension generates distension and protrusion of the lamellae of the annulus much more than in flexion. From Adams et al., 1988 [16], with permission

substantial impact on the annulus. Conversely, in a disc with even initial degenerative phenomena, extension generates a posterior protrusion of the annulus that can be very marked, while flexion generates a minimal anterior protrusion.

Along the same lines, another study using MRI on healthy subjects studied the displacement of the nucleus during lateral flexion [18]. The study argues for an internal displacement of the nucleus towards the convexity, but paradoxically, the images also show an evident external protrusion of the annulus towards the concavity.

In summary, during flexion, the nucleus of a healthy disc tends to protrude, more by deformation than by translation, towards the convexity. At the same time, the elastic tension of the posterior annulus is maintained, which resists well even if shortened in extension. On the contrary, in a disc with even very initial degeneration, the nucleus constantly protrudes from the part of the concavity because it finds less resistance in a less resistant (because it is damaged or "flaccid" due to inelasticity). In any case, the protrusion is mainly due to the annulus and not the nucleus. On the other hand, disc degeneration involves dehydration of the nucleus (whose mass, therefore, tends to reduce) and not only less elastic resistance to the distension of the annulus.

6.1.3   The Yellow Ligaments: Not to be Overlooked

We must not limit ourselves to considering disc protrusion to formulate a compressive model of low back pain. It is essential to consider the overall section of the vertebral canal to which compressive and ischemic suffering of the algogenic structures can be traced. The section can also be reduced posteriorly by the yellow ligaments and the interapophyseal joints (or "facets"), as in the narrow canal syndrome.

As mentioned, the yellow ligaments connect the laminae of adjacent vertebrae and are rich in elastin. It is not uncommon to find a radiological finding of "hypertrophy" of the yellow ligaments attributable to fibrosis and fatty deposits and an expression of a typical degenerative process. However, it should be remembered that even in intact spines, the yellow ligaments are subject to protrude inside the vertebral canal posteriorly in case of extension of the lumbar spine, as demonstrated by multiple anatomical and in vivo studies [19–22].

6.1.4 The "Facet Syndrome" ("Facet Joint Syndrome")

Since the works of Mixter and Barr (see also in Frymoyer [23]), it has been recognised that the interapophyseal joints ("facets") easily undergo arthritic deformities in parallel with the reduction in disc thickness. Sometimes, they can also emit synovial cysts that cause direct radicular compression. In addition to generating joint pain, the phenomenon, characterised by osteophytic production, can contribute significantly to canal stenosis, particularly foraminal stenosis, or stenosis of one or both conjugation foramina from which the roots emerge. As mentioned several times, the cross-section of the vertebral canal then takes on the already mentioned "trefoil" shape.

Many therapeutic proposals emphasise the role of facets as at least a relevant, if not sufficient, source of lumbosciatic pain. For a review on the subject, see Du et al. [24] and Cohen and Raja [25]. Semi-invasive forms of diagnosis (anaesthetic infiltration RX- or echo-guided) and physical therapy (sensory denervation with radio frequencies) or surgical (facetectomy) are often used. In truth, it is somewhat doubtful that this approach can lead to more than temporary benefits since facet arthrosis is just one of the many signs of degeneration of the vertebral disc complex.

6.1.5 Spondylolisthesis and "Instability" in Chronic Low Back Pain

It is not uncommon to observe on the sagittal plane a modest "slippage" (listhesis, from ancient Greek "olísthesis": see note on page 23, Chap. 2) of a lumbar vertebra anterior to the one below. More rarely, the slippage is posterior. Imaging reports (radiography, CT, MRI) usually place a lot of emphasis on this finding. In the absence of a bilateral spondylolysis that disconnects the vertebral body from the arch, the "slippage" reflects a deformation of the facets and a lack of hold of the longitudinal and yellow ligaments. Once again, it is a sign of degeneration of the vertebro-disc complex. In axial CT or MRI projection, the anterior slippage leaves the posterior portion of the disc exposed, thus giving a false image of hernia. The vertebral canal, therefore, may be wider than normal. Spondylolisthesis is considered a suspected cause of "intervertebral instability", for which confirmation is sought with "functional" radiographic projections in statics and maximum flexion and extension of the trunk (much more rarely with MRI on dedicated instruments). Most instability diagnoses, however, occur on arthritic columns even without evidence of spondylolisthesis. I share the many opinions accumulated over the decades, according to which a modest spondylolisthesis is essentially harmless, and the existence of an "instability" syndrome is at least doubtful [15, 26–29].

Consider that the diagnosis of lumbar instability can lead to somewhat invasive stabilisation interventions with arthrodesis and metal synthesis (fusion) and that the "block" of two or more vertebrae risks leading within a few years to compensatory hypermobility (and symptomatic) of the adjacent vertebrae, as will be seen later. Therefore, the indication for "stabilisation" interventions, which will be recalled later, remains controversial [30].

6.1.6 The Overall Section of the Vertebral Canal in Flexion and Extension

A Swedish radiologist [31] is credited with the first systematic study on anatomical samples and then with in vivo myelography of the section of the lumbar vertebral canal and its variations in flexion-extension movements. Subsequent studies with MRI in asymptomatic subjects [19] or with narrow canal syndrome [32] have confirmed his elegant results. In particular, this last study provided the dimensions of the lumbar vertebral canal in subjects with canal stenosis. The transverse area of the canal increased by 20%, and the anteroposterior diameter by 10% in flexion, compared to what happened in extension (the area and the anteroposterior diameter were minimal at the L4/L5 level. As I have already mentioned, in my experience, it is more common to observe symptomatic stenosis on the L3 or even L2 level).

Therefore, it is easy to imagine how in a canal affected by stenosis, but also in a normal canal placed in extension, the extension itself may cause a narrowing critical for the roots of the cauda (and for its vessels, as discussed above). This aspect has been overlooked by much of the literature on lumbosciatic pain. This literature has been much more interested in the intra-discal mechanics and disc-radicular conflicts than in the overall dynamics of the canal section. It is evident, however, that a disc protrusion will have very different clinical effects depending on the section of the canal towards which it protrudes. In practice, the lumbar extension will result in a compression of the contents of the spine for two reasons: the posterior protrusion of the annulus and the reduction in the transverse area of the vertebral canal. To complete the picture, however, a key player in the content of the vertebral canal, namely the dural sac, is still missing.

6.1.7 The Mechanics of the Dural Sac

The dural sac (or dura mater, dura meninge, or "dura") wraps the central nervous system and the roots of the cauda. At the level of the conjugation foramina, the sac is extruded with sheaths that accompany the roots, merging then with the epineurium. Very noticeable dural cysts often form at the sacral level in MRI (Tarlov's cysts). These cysts are harmless and do not cause pain.

At the lumbar level, as already mentioned, the dural sac is innervated by the recurrent meningeal nerves of Luschka, a reference to which has been made previously. It is well known that an irritated dura (for example, in septic or aseptic meningitis) generates intense pain.

It is worth repeating here that, as in all serous membranes (peritoneum, pericardium, pleura, joint synovia), the innervation of the dura is not easily attributable to a precise radicular level. In the course of the development of these structures, the original metamerism, well present in the muscles and the sensory-somatic dermatomeria, is lost. In the case of the dural sac, things get complicated by the particular course of the Luschka nerves, which intersect and extend in cranial and caudal branches, thus losing a strict connection with their level of entrance into the spinal canal. However, when the suffering site is considered, the mechanism that accentuates pain becomes much more straightforward: stretching the dural sac. This can occur by flexing the head, flexing the dorsal or lumbar spine, and stretching the nerves of the lower limbs. The stretching of a nerve (for example, the sciatic nerve) is transmitted to the roots that compose it and to their dural sheaths (typically, in the Lasègue sign). Therefore, lumbar pain of dural origin is easily recognised because the patient prefers a hyperlordotic position (see Fig. 1.1 and the paragraph on the "extensor" patient).

References

1. Nachemson A, Morris JM. In vivo intradiscal pressure measurement: discometry, a method for determining pressure in the lower lumbar discs. J Bone Joint Surg. 1964;46-A(5):1077–91.
2. Wilke HJ, Neef P, Hinz B, Seidel H, Claes L. Intradiscal pressure together with anthropometric data - a data set for the validation of models. Clin Biomech. 2001;16(Suppl. No. 1):S111–26.
3. Li JQ, Kwong WH, Chan YL, Kawabata M. Comparison of in vivo intradiscal pressure between sitting and standing in human lumbar spine: a systematic review and meta-analysis. Life. 2022;12(3):457.
4. Brown T, Hansen RJ, Yorra AJ. Some mechanical tests on the lumbosacral spine, with particular reference to the intervertebral discs: a preliminary report. J Bone Joint Surg. 1957;39(5):1135–64.
5. McKenzie R, May S. The lumbar spine mechanical diagnosis & therapy. 2nd ed. Wellington: Spinal Publications; 2003.
6. Fennell AJ, Jones AP, Hukins DW. Migration of the nucleus pulposus within the intervertebral disc during spine flexion and extension. Spine. 1996;21(23):2753–7.
7. Brault JS, Driscoll DM, Laakso L, Kappler RE, Allin EF, Glonek T. Quantification of lumbar intradiscal deformation during flexion and extension, by mathematical analysis of magnetic resonance imaging pixel intensity profiles. Spine. 1997;22(18):2066–72.
8. Schnebel BE, Simmons JW, Chowning J, Davidson R. A digitising technique for the study of movement. Spine. 1988;13(3):309–12.
9. Penning L, Wilmink J. Biomechanics of lumbosacral dural sac. A study of flexion-extension myelography. Spine. 1981;6(4):398–408.
10. Edmondston SJ, Song S, Bricknell RV, Davies PA, Fersum K, Humphries P, et al. MRI evaluation of lumbar spine flexion and extension in asymptomatic individuals. Man Ther. 2000;5(3):158–64.

11. Parent EC, Videman T, Battié MC. The effect of lumbar flexion and extension on disc contour abnormality was measured quantitatively on magnetic resonance imaging. Spine. 2006;31(24):2836–42.

12. Zou J, Yang H, Miyazaki M, Morishita Y, Wei F, Mcgovern S, et al. Dynamic bulging of intervertebral discs in the degenerative lumbar spine. Spine. 2009;34(23):2545–50.

13. Lao LF, Zhong GB, Li QY, Liu ZD. Kinetic magnetic resonance imaging analysis of spinal degeneration: a systematic review. Orthop Surg. 2014;6(4):294–9.

14. Jinkins JR, Dworkin JS, Damadian RV. Upright, weight-bearing, dynamic-kinetic MRI of the spine: initial results. Eur Radiol. 2005;15(9):1815–25.

15. Michelini G, Corridore A, Torlone S, Bruno F, Marsecano C, Capasso R, et al. Dynamic MRI in the evaluation of the spine: state of the art. Acta Biomed. 2018;89(1-S):89–101.

16. Adams MA, Dolan P, Hutton WC. The lumbar spine in backward bending. Spine. 1988;13(9):1019–26.

17. Nazari J, Pope MH, Graveling RA. Reality about migration of the nucleus pulposus within the intervertebral disc with changing postures. Clin Biomech. 2012;27(3):213–7.

18. Fazey PJ, Takasaki H, Singer KP. Nucleus pulposus deformation in response to lumbar spine lateral flexion: an in vivo MRI investigation. Eur Spine J. 2010;19(7):1115–20.

19. Schmid MR, Stucki G, Duewell S, Wildermuth S, Romanowski B, Hodler J. Changes in cross-sectional measurements of the spinal canal and intervertebral foramina as a function of body position: in vivo studies on an open-configuration MR system. Am J Roentgenol. 1999;172:1095–102.

20. Inufusa A, An HS, Lim TY, Hasegawa T, Haughton V, Novicki B. Anatomic changes of the spinal canal and intervertebral foramen associated with flexion-extension movement. Spine. 1996;21(21):2412–20.

21. Chung SS, Lee CS, Kim SH, Kim SH, Chung MW, Ann JM. Effect of low back posture on the morphology of the spinal canal. Skeletal Radiol. 2000;29:217–23.

22. Ho PSP, Yu S, Sether LA, Wagner M, Ho KC, Haughton VM. Ligamentum flavum: appearance on sagittal and coronal MR images. Radiology. 1988;168:469–72.

23. Frymoyer JW. Back pain and sciatica. N Engl J Med. 1988;31:291–300.

24. Du R, Xu G, Bai X, Li Z. Facet joint syndrome: pathophysiology, diagnosis, and treatment. J Pain Res. 2022;15:3689–710.

25. Cohen SP, Raja SN. Pathogenesis, diagnosis, and treatment of lumbar zygapophysial (facet) joint pain. Anesthesiology. 2007;106(3):591–614.

26. Stokes IA, Frymoyer JW. Segmental motion and instability. Spine. 1987;12(7):688–91.

27. Mitchell UH, Hurrell J. Clinical spinal instability: 10 years since the derivation of a clinical prediction rule. A narrative literature review. J Back Musculoskelet Rehabil. 2019;32:293–8.

28. Fritz JM, Erhard RE, Hagen BF. Segmental instability of the lumbar spine. Phys Ther. 1998;78(8):889–96.

29. Leone A, Cassar-Pullicino VN, Guglielmi G, Bonomo L. Degenerative lumbar intervertebral instability: what is it and how does imaging contribute? Skeletal Radiol. 2009;38:529–33.

30. Harris IA, Traeger A, Stanford R, Maher CG, Buchbinder R. Lumbar spine fusion: what is the evidence? Intern Med J. 2018;48(12):1430–4.

31. Knutsson F. Volume and shape variations of the vertebral canal in lordosis and kyphosis and their significance for the myelographic diagnosis. Acta Radiol. 1942;23(5):431–43.

32. Kanbara S, Yukawa Y, Ito K, Machino M, Kato F. Dynamic changes in the dural sac of patients with lumbar canal stenosis evaluated by multidetector-row computed tomography after myelography. Eur Spine J. 2014;23(1):74–9.

7.1 Why the Flexor Picture: Non-meningeal Compression

At this point in the discussion, many apparent inconsistencies in the clinical picture of chronic lower back pain should be placed in a rational pathogenetic frame. The flexed position of the lumbar spine alleviates pain simply because it widens the canal. Any form of compression (disc, osteophytic, venous) is consequently attenuated.

7.2 Why the Extensor Picture: Meningeal Irritation

The paragraph on the mechanics of the dural sac explains well why some patients prefer a hyperextended position: the section of the vertebral canal is reduced, but the meningeal pain, which has priority, is attenuated. Nothing prevents the patient from suffering in an extended position if the relaxation of the dural sac is insufficient or if a compressive mechanism is accentuated. As already mentioned, it is not uncommon for the "extensor" patient, typically suffering from very acute pain, once the "meningeal phase" is resolved, to transform into a more typical flexor patient with chronic pain.

7.3 Pain at Rest

Venous dilation explains the pain accentuated by rest (but more generally by prolonged postures). It is well known that standing still for a long time may cause "swollen feet" due to venous stasis and consequent oedema.

The Batson plexus, in particular, lacks actual valves. In the absence of a muscular pump, therefore, it dilates quickly. This explains the typical condition of morning stiffness. Consider what many patients report, that the worst moment of the day

© The Author(s), under exclusive license to Springer Nature
Switzerland AG 2025

L. Tesio, *Low Back Pain and Sciatica*,
https://doi.org/10.1007/978-3-031-78534-4_7

is when they bend over the sink to brush their teeth or, even worse, in the case of men, to shave: the increase in disc pressure connected to the contraction of the paravertebral muscles finds a very unfavourable context in the venous stasis accumulated during the night. The pain mechanism during or immediately after rest is familiar to sinusitis, osteomyelitis, and dental pulpitis, involving venous dilation in restricted bone spaces.

7.4   Pain in Pregnancy

Understanding the role of the epidural venous plexus as an 'escape route' in pregnancy-related pain is a significant part of our knowledge in this field. The pain usually increases during hours of rest, even during the day. In a static position, a hyperlordotic position is needed to move back the body's centre of mass, unbalanced forward by the weight of the gravid uterus.

7.5   Risk Factors

The rheumatological studies of the Jayson school (see Chap. 5) convincingly explain why a fibrinolytic deficit can be associated with lower back pain, especially if it is chronic. Post-phlebitic epidural fibrosis is facilitated not only by venous stasis but also by possible thrombophilia: this is why cardiovascular diseases and low back pain share risk factors such as smoking, obesity, dyslipidemia, and a sedentary lifestyle.

7.6   Radicular Signs that Disappear: Algogenic Inhibition More than Radicular Damage

It has already been said that patients with lower back pain or sciatic or crural pain who present frank radicular signs (reduced or abolished tendon reflexes; hypoesthesia; strength deficit) are relatively rare. When there are, these signs usually do not indicate radicular damage (neither axonal nor demyelinating) but an algogenic inhibition connected to referred pain. The inhibition extends to thermoregulatory control. The patient often reports feeling cold feet. Cutaneous hypothermia with radicular distribution is observed (even 2–3° less on the skin of the foot on the painful side compared to the contralateral foot). It is well described that the fact that somatic pain can cause hypoesthesia, hypotonia, abolition of tendon reflexes, and hypothermia: all signs that can quickly recede if the pain subsides [1–3]. Therefore, the most worrying neurological signs are those that do not associate with pain or do not normalise when the pain disappears. This is mainly true for strength deficits.

Nevertheless, in my experience, sensory symptoms (hypoesthesia/dysesthesia with radicular distribution) and tendon hyporeflexia can persist much longer for reasons that are not entirely known (direct suffering of the sensory ganglion or the sensory root as from actual radicular axonal damage?). It should be remembered that electromyographic examination has little usefulness despite being prescribed very frequently. Even in chronic situations, when modest signs of motor unit remodelling are the rule, normal sensory conduction is expected on electromyographic testing because the compression on sensitive fibres, if any, is pre-ganglionic (the trophic centre remains intact).

It should also be reiterated that foot weakness (more frequently in dorsal than plantar flexion) should be carefully monitored, primarily if not associated with intense pain. Apart from causes independent of the lumbar spine (initial motor neuron diseases, for example), a potent strength loss may reveal significant axonal compression (and not central inhibition) and, therefore, a prelude to paralysing sciatica as already described.

7.7   Persistence of Results with Mechanical Therapies

This point will be addressed later. However, suppose one succeeds in fostering the venous outflow (with the methods described in Chap. 2). In that case, one can hope for a definitive resolution of the phlebitic processes that usually accompany the narrowing of the vertebral canal section. The canal narrowing results in stasis and increased venous pressure, but we can aim for a positive outcome with the right approach.

7.8   Why Lumbar Pain Instead of Radiated or Referred Pain

The interapophyseal joints (facets), the annulus, the posterior longitudinal ligament, and the epidural veins can produce a typical nociceptive pain localised in the lumbar area approximately at the lesion level.

The compression/inflammation of the sensitive roots (or the spinal ganglion) generates radiated pain with root distribution (this is typical for intra or extraforaminal disc herniations or osteophytes that protrude into the conjugation foramina). This is not the case for meningeal pain, which, as mentioned, generates a much less precise "reference" at both the lumbar level and the lower limbs, usually without extending beyond the thigh, and can be associated with neurovegetative disorders (typically nausea). All these distributions underlie a common pathogenetic mechanism, and nothing prevents them from coexisting in the individual case.

7.9   Spontaneous Healing, Recurring Episodes, Chronicity

It is well known that lumbar pain can usually disappear spontaneously within 6 weeks [4]. If this duration is exceeded, the possibility of spontaneous healing rapidly decreases but remains possible. The CT or MRI picture can remain unchanged in all these cases: an apparent paradox. The pathogenetic model is much more complex than the compression one. Firstly, connective and nerve structures can adapt by becoming more extensible and experience lower strains for the same elongation. Secondly, the nucleus pulposus tends to dehydrate over time. The "disappearance" of even bulky disc herniations within months or years is not rare [5]. Thirdly, a venous-phlebitic component already has a good chance of spontaneous resolution if the fibrinolytic mechanisms slowly manage to resolve local fibrosis: anyone who has suffered from haemorrhoids or lower limb phlebitis knows that these diseases can also resolve themselves with a bit of patience.

The onset of pain, its resolution, its recurrences or the chronicization all reflect a very individual pathogenesis based on high-level and personal interactions between osteoarticular, venous, and inflammatory factors. The "compressive" simplification of pathogenesis and excessive confidence in imaging generate paradoxes that are not such. In addition, in many cases, compressive pictures (for disc herniation or stenosis) are entirely asymptomatic. If they become so, this is due to concurrent causes that fade away. Therefore, treating chronic low back pain does not necessarily mean restoring an anatomy that appears altered to us, and that was probably so for a long time before the symptoms manifested. Treating the patient means taking a small step back towards a completely asymptomatic context.

References

1. Knutsson E, Skoglund CR, Natchev E. Changes in voluntary muscle strength, somatosensory transmission and skin temperature concomitant with pain relief during autotraction in patients with lumbar and sacral root lesions. Pain. 1988;33(2):173–9.
2. Stokes M, Young A. The contribution of reflex inhibition to arthrogenous muscle weakness. Clin Sci. 1984;67:7–14.
3. Callaghan MJ, Parkes MJ, Hutchinson CE, Felson DT. Factors associated with arthrogenous muscle inhibition in patellofemoral osteoarthritis. Osteoarthr Cartil. 2014;22(6):742–6.
4. Frymoyer JW. Back pain and sciatica. N Engl J Med. 1988;31:291–300.
5. Komori H, Shinomiya K, Nakai O, Yamaura I, Takeda S, Furuya K. The natural history of herniated nucleus pulposus with radiculopathy. Spine. 1996;21(2):225–9.

Part IV

An Integrated Pathogenetic Model and Some Particular Cases

The Compressive-Venous-Inflammatory Model

8

The pathogenetic model that I propose here, the CoVIn model, is consistent with all the observations reported above. It considers an interaction between compressive, venous vascular, and inflammatory factors. This model has significant implications for clinical practice, as it provides a comprehensive understanding of chronic lumbosciatic pain. Figure 8.1 schematises the model, offering a visual aid for its application in practice.

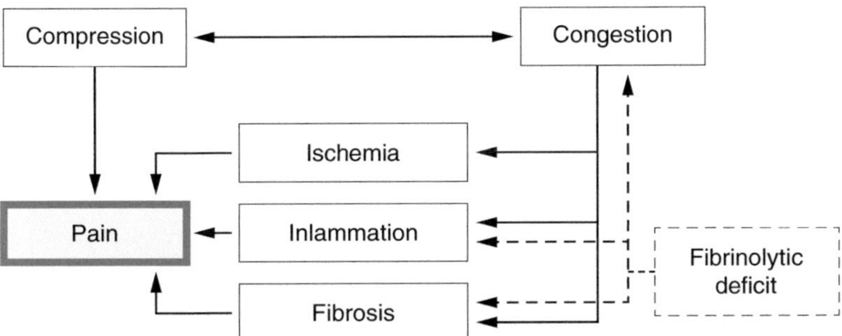

Fig. 8.1 The CoVIn pathogenetic model of benign chronic lumbosciatic pain

© The Author(s), under exclusive license to Springer Nature Switzerland AG 2025
L. Tesio, *Low Back Pain and Sciatica*,
https://doi.org/10.1007/978-3-031-78534-4_8

8.1   Model Synthesis

In the CoVIn model, pain originates from compression of algogenic nerve endings (inflamed roots, ganglia, sensitive ligaments, vascular or meningeal nerve fibres) by various anatomical structures (disc, joints, yellow ligaments and others). The epidural venous system (Batson's plexus) can quickly dilate and add compression but also produce ischemia and epidural phlebitic inflammation. The latter can become chronic, evolving into fibrosis, especially if fibrinolysis is deficient: a condition facilitated by underlying metabolic risk factors (smoking, diabetes, dyslipidemia, sedentary lifestyle). Fibrosis incarcerates epidural but also intradural nerve endings, sometimes even the spinal roots, and becomes a source of chronic pain. As a rule, enlarging the vertebral canal through lumbar flexion provides relief. Still, suppose the compressive-inflammatory phenomenon involves the dural sac. In that case, the spine extension will provide relief because, while reducing the section of the vertebral canal, it will allow the dural sac to be relaxed. The model was presented in a recent article [1].

8.2   How and What the Model Explains

Figure 8.2 summarises how the model explains the eight contradictions listed in Table 1.1 and taken up in the boxes on the left.

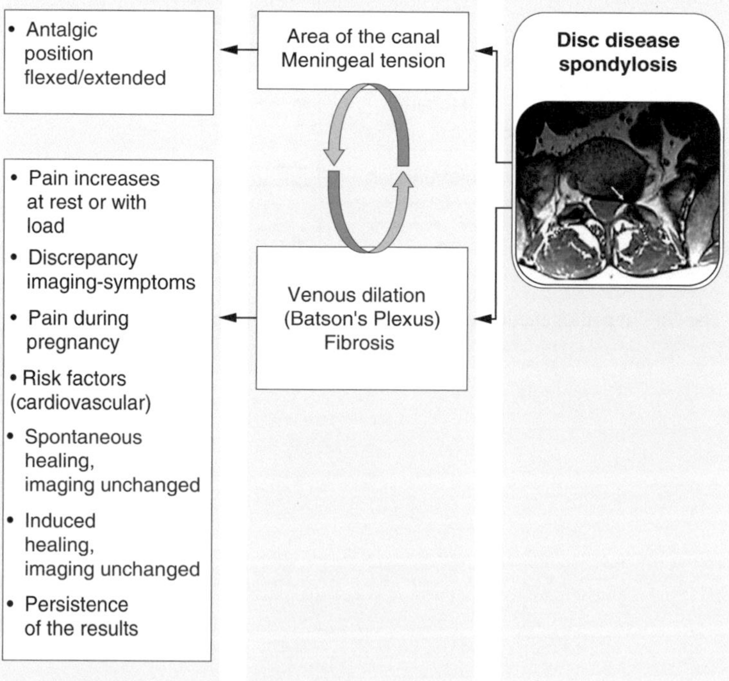

Fig. 8.2 Relationship between apparent contradictions in "low back pain" pictures and components of the CoVIn model

The compressive component and that of traction on the dural sac (central panel) explain the preference for the flexed or extended position; the dilation of the veins belonging to the Batson plexus and the possible phlebitic-fibrotic evolution explains all the other contradictions. Ultimately, the three mechanisms (compressive, venous and phlebitic-inflammatory) can be traced back to a single degenerative pathology of the disc-vertebral complex (recalled by the image on the right). However, in individual cases, the predominance of one or the other mechanism and the different interactions between the mechanisms, reported in Fig. 8.1, may give rise to multiple behavioural manifestations, multiple forms of pain and various responses to different conservative therapies.

Based on the CoVIn model, I will now demonstrate how it can be applied to understand particular cases of chronic lumbosciatic pain. Hopefully, this practical application will enable clinicians to make informed decisions about prescribing conservative treatment, enhancing their ability to manage this complex condition effectively.

8.3   A Pragmatic Proposal: From "Lumbosciatica" to "CoVin Lumbosciatica"

However, before closing this chapter, it is worth asking whether the acronym CoViN can be introduced into clinical practice.

Let's look at the typical patients who come to the clinic: overall, dozens or hundreds of times a year. As a rule, the patient is an adult between 40 and 65 years old with lumbar or lumbosciatic pain for many weeks, arising primarily upon waking or sitting for a long time, especially in the following standing up. Walking and even lifting weights with a minimum of caution does not increase the pain. Medications do little; the various physical analgesic therapies are even less effective. MRI and CT scans of the lumbar spine often show modest disc protrusions and initial facet joint arthritis. X-rays do not reveal anything correlated with the pain itself. The EMG shows nonspecific radicular signs in the legs, without sensory or motor deficit. The Lasègue sign is negative. The patient prefers to stay with the trunk flexed. Extending the lumbar column causes discomfort and sometimes intense pain.

This patient should no longer be labelled as a case of "low back pain", and that's it: now he could be classified as a case of CoVIn low back pain or a case of benign compressive-venous-inflammatory lumbar disorder that certainly manifests with pain but also with reductions in mobility and alterations in the posture of the trunk. If we listen to the acronym, relieving pain is no longer the immediate goal: the goal becomes to create space within the vertebral canal by acting on the joint and disc mechanics, as well as the epidural venous stasis.

This variation of the diagnostic coding, from descriptive to pathophysiological based on knowledge progress, is certainly not new in Medicine. For example, the old "calcific scapulohumeral periarthritis" has long since become a syndrome of acromion-clavicular muscle impingement [2]. Many signs and symptoms localised to the foot (hallux valgus, plantar fasciitis, "flatness" of the arch, Achilles bursitis, "claw" fingers, calluses, Morton's inter-metatarsal neuroma, etc.), in variable combinations, are now framed as elements of a shared "pronation syndrome": and this thanks to the fundamental studies of Merton L. Root that have allowed to trace almost all these disorders back to a congenital alteration of the talus-calcaneus orientation [3].

Therefore, describing the patient as a "case of CoVIn low back pain" signals a greater pathophysiological understanding of the clinical picture and provides a structured approach to treatment. This can help caregivers avoid a hasty choice of purely symptomatic pain therapies, ensuring patients receive the most effective and appropriate care.

References

1. Tesio L. Low back pain: a new comprehensive pathogenetic model supports methods of Medical Rehabilitation. Bull Rehabil Med. 2023;22(5):83–92.
2. Creech JA, Silver S. Shoulder impingement syndrome [updated 2023 Apr 17]. In: StatPearls [Internet]. Treasure Island, FL: StatPearls Publishing, 2024 Jan. Available from: https://www.ncbi.nlm.nih.gov/books/NBK554518/.
3. Root ML, Orien WP, Weed JH. Normal and abnormal function of the foot. Vol II. Clinical Biomechanics Corp. , Los Angeles, CA-USA, 1977: pp.1–478.

Cases that Are Compatible with the CoVln Model

9.1 Post-surgical Cases

9.1.1 Premise

Physiatrists (but I believe the same can be said of neurologists, rheumatologists, pain therapy specialists, and family doctors) see many patients with lower back pain unresolved by surgical interventions; consequently, they have a distorted, pessimistic view of the effectiveness of surgery on lumbosciatic pain. The troubled stories of these patients include an endless and not always rational series of unsuccessful conservative approaches: the war between proponents of conservative approaches and proponents of surgical techniques, therefore, is often a war between the poor. The war is fueled by a pathophysiological knowledge (to which this book would like to contribute) that, due to its incompleteness, ends up justifying the most varied, arbitrary and often imaginative treatments and, ultimately, the choice for the "last resort" surgery.

9.1.2 Surgery, Not Always the Right Solution: It Doesn't Always Work

It's important to remember that surgical interventions in cases of lumbosciatalgia are very frequent and, for the vast majority, effective. This text does not want to discuss their indications. However, the importance of conservative treatments— mechanical or pharmacological—before planning an operation cannot be overemphasised. Patients usually prefer the conservative solution, but no two patients have followed the same path. Knowledge empowers physicians to make informed decisions in their practice.

When patients arrive at the point of considering surgery, they often do so after numerous, extensive, and costly conservative attempts. This underscores the

© The Author(s), under exclusive license to Springer Nature Switzerland AG 2025

L. Tesio, *Low Back Pain and Sciatica*, https://doi.org/10.1007/978-3-031-78534-4_9

importance of Medicine being guided by pathophysiological knowledge that is as solid as possible (the goal of this book). Such knowledge should rationalise the decision to resort to surgery in the event of conservative treatment failure.

Remember that it is not rare for a patient to present to the doctor after an operation that has not had satisfactory results. The most common case is that of the patient operated on for disc herniation. Today, the operation is usually based on microsurgery, which, when things go well, allows the resumption of daily activities after a few days [1, 2].

9.1.3 Instability and "Surgical Stabilisation": A Controversial Rationale

There are also patients operated on for laminectomy, hemilaminectomy or foraminotomy for narrow lumbar canal and patients who have undergone more invasive "stabilisation" (fusion) interventions of two or more lumbar vertebrae, possibly "fused" also with the sacrum. It has already been said that the concept of "instability" is at least controversial. The "stabilisation" (which has already been mentioned) follows the most varied techniques and is essentially based on the application of metal synthesis (inter-peduncular screws and plates) and vertebral spacers or vertebral arthrodesis (autologous bone graft, interbody metal cages). All interventions on the lumbar spine present a risk - between 1% and 5% - of acute or subacute surgical complications (dural fistula, epidural hematoma, radicular lesion, infection) [3]. Stabilisation, however, also involves specific risks related to non-fusion, mobilisation or incorrect positioning of the screws. It is important to remember, then, the early arthro-discal degeneration of the level immediately cranial to the stabilisation itself, which becomes subject to compensatory hyper-mobility and possibly disc herniation (so-called adjacent segment degeneration, ASD) [4].

In my experience, "adjacent" should be understood flexibly. It is not uncommon to see disc herniations (even rare ones, like those of the first and second lumbar discs) develop two or more segments above those stabilised. The time of appearance can vary from a few months to 5–10 years after the surgical intervention.

Figure 9.1 refers to an exemplary case of chronic lower back pain treated with stabilisation (interpeduncular screws and plates at L4 and L5 levels and intersomatic spacer). After about 8 months of well-being, intense lower back pain appeared. The appearance of disc protrusions (not present in a preoperative MRI) at the three levels above stabilisation is evident.

Figure 9.2 refers to another exemplary case of adjacent segment degeneration. The patient suffered from continuous lumbosciatic pain with pain referred to the right buttock and the posterolateral face of the right thigh. The patient had been operated on 10 years earlier for removal of the fifth lumbar disc hernia and stabilisation with only interpeduncular screws L5-S1 (one on the right and one on the left), without benefit. In the last 6 months, the patient has reported a marked worsening of the lower back pain that has forced him to reduce walking to a few tens of meters

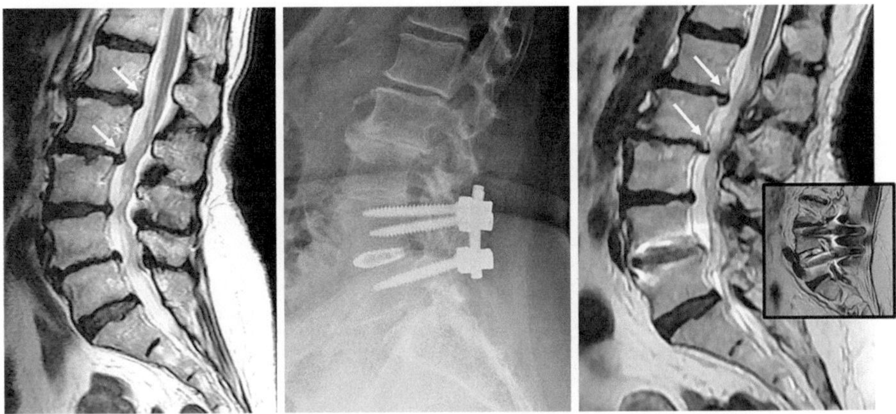

Fig. 9.1 75-year-old woman with low back pain and intense left inguinal pain for 4 months. Five years earlier, the patient had undergone surgical stabilisation (interpeduncular screws at level L4-L5 and inter-somatic spacer) with good immediate results. On the left: preoperative sagittal MRI image of the lumbar spine. In the centre: postoperative sagittal RX image that clearly shows the surgical inserts. On the right is a recent sagittal MRI image. The small insert shows a picture taken from the same examination, indirectly highlighting the screws. A moderate increase in a pre-existing L2/L3 protrusion and a marked increase in an L1/L2 disc protrusion (white arrows in the MRI images) are visible and compatible with the site of inguinal pain. Personal observation

and to use a cane. A current MRI shows a L5/S1 disc hernia (recurrence?) and especially a new L2/L3 disc hernia.

9.1.4   Repeated Surgical Interventions

For herniectomy (the most frequent intervention), the rate of symptomatic recurrence is around 3–5% in the following 5 years. In general, a re-intervention has less chance of clinical success because, inevitably, the first intervention leaves epidural scars that are in themselves a potential source of pain. In general, the risk increases further if the intervention, as may be necessary, consists of a combination of different procedures and if the repeated interventions are more than one.

It's important to understand and empathize with patients who have been operated on several times and who present the so-called 'failed back syndrome'. This term represents a euphemism. The failure does not concern the lumbar spine but the surgeon: not necessarily due to his operative demerit but sometimes due to incorrect indication [5, 6]. However, the definition effectively summarises a picture consisting of chronic lower back or lumbosciatic pain, often tormenting, supported mainly by epidural fibrosis and possibly by hernia recurrences not easily operable in the new context.

Almost all cases of lower back or sciatic pain that persists even at a distance from the surgical intervention fall within the CoVIn model and precisely (when the

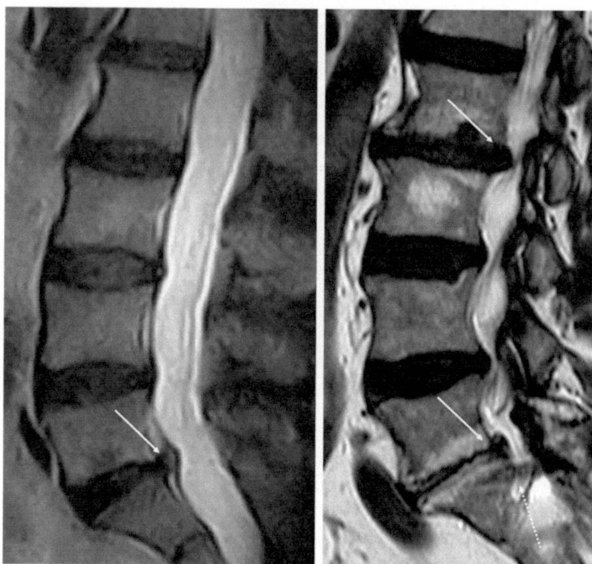

Fig. 9.2 Lumbar MRI before and after L5/S1 stabilisation—72-year-old man with lumbosciatica. For years, he suffered from intense right lumbosciatic pain worsened in the last 6 months. Ten years earlier, the patient had undergone surgery to remove a hernia from the fifth lumbar disc and stabilisation with interpeduncular screws (right and left) L5/S1. There has never been a substantial benefit. The image on the left (lumbar MRI with sagittal cut) shows the preoperative picture: a sub-ligamentous L5/S1 hernia (arrow) is visible. The postoperative picture is represented by the MRI image on the right. A screw is indirectly recognisable (dashed white arrow). A recurrent L5/S1 hernia (continuous arrow at the bottom) is noted, consistent with the pain referred to the lower limb. The subchondral oedema of the adjacent vertebral plates L5 and S1 is also very evident (more apparent than in the other vertebral bodies). There is also the appearance of a disc herniation at the L2/L3 level (white arrow at the top), consistent with intense lower back pain (personal observation)

spine's mobility allows it) in the above-defined "flexor" picture. In cases of recurrent hernia or residual pain post-laminectomy, all the pathophysiological considerations expressed so far apply, with the addition that the role of venous stasis and a more or less latent epidural phlebitis underlying the inevitable scar fibrosis can be considered increased.

The case of pain that persists or appears months or years after stabilisation is different. It is not uncommon for the dissatisfied patient to reappear to the surgeon who, observing recent images, responds that "the intervention went well" and that "plates and screws are in place": a dialogue between deaf people. The patient is interested in the pain, and the surgeon is interested in the correctly position of the metal synthesis. In my experience, the pain is almost always underpinned by ASD, as mentioned earlier, or by early discarthrosis pathology in a segment above the stabilisation. Furthermore, misfortune upon misfortune, even in the stabilised segments, a symptomatic disc protrusion may manifest itself that must be sought with MRI, despite some inevitable artefacts also with MRI-compatible synthesis means.

Perhaps little can be done to cure the pain. However, an anatomical explanation is still essential to avoid the patient receiving the blaming label of "psychiatric" (a topic that will be addressed in Chap. 10). As a rule, these patients are disappointed, become depressed and eventually migrate to pain therapy centres (see below) or turn to "alternative" medicines [7], resigning themselves to the incurability of their clinical picture.

Surgical solutions may exist, including removing all or part of the synthesis, which means starting the case from scratch. Few surgeons - understandably - readily admit clinical failure in the presence of an anatomical "success"; above all, many fear - rightly - adding further complications to a case in which the patient is expected to be demanding. There is room for pathophysiological mechanical treatment with techniques focused on epidural venous decongestion. Mobilisation exercises would only increase the hypermobility of the segments adjacent to those operated on. For this reason, I recommend active lumbar traction in the supine or side position, but without mobilisation of the spine or water exercise, techniques that will be the subject of dedicated paragraphs. Even mild fibrinolytic therapy appears to be a rational option, as will be seen later.

References

1. Dowling TJ, Munakomi S, Dowling TJ. Microdiskectomy. In: StatPearls [Internet]. Treasure Island, FL: StatPearls Publishing; 2023.
2. Postacchini F, Postacchini R. Operative management of lumbar disc herniation: the evolution of knowledge and surgical techniques in the last century. Acta Neurochir Suppl. 2011;108:17–21.
3. Willson MC, Ross JS. Postoperative spine complications. Neuroimaging Clin N Am. 2014;24(2):305–26.
4. Sakaura H, Ikegami D, Fuji T. Early cephalad adjacent segment degeneration after posterior lumbar interbody fusion: a comparative study between cortical bone trajectory screw fixation and traditional trajectory screw fixation. J Neurosurg. 2019;32(2):155–9.
5. Baber Z, Erdek MA. Failed back surgery syndrome: current perspectives. J Pain Res. 2016;9:979–87.
6. Nachemson A. Failed back surgery syndrome is a syndrome of failed back surgeons. Pain Clin. 1999;11(4):271–84.
7. Tesio L. Alternative medicines: yes; alternatives to medicine: no. Am J Phys Med Rehabil. 2013;92(6):542–5.

Cases at the Boundaries or Outside the CoVIn Model

10.1 Lower Back or Sciatic Pain in Bone Deformity of the Spine

10.1.1 Pain in Idiopathic or Acquired Scoliosis

Lower back and/or sciatic pain can afflict patients with spinal deformities due to either idiopathic scoliosis or neuromuscular diseases (for example, outcomes of poliomyelitis, spinal amyotrophy, and myopathies). It should be stated that the scoliotic deformity itself does not explain the pain. These cases also fall within the CoVIn model - flexor framework. Typically, the pain appears decades after the onset of the disease when the deformity is stabilised. The spinal cord, roots, muscles, and ligaments have had time to adapt, but everything is limited.

The articular facets typically develop arthritic deformities from overload and generate stenosis. Often, it is unilateral foraminal stenosis: the exit path of the roots from the spine is blocked. Lordosis gives bilateral stenosis. Conversely, the concavity and torsion of the spine give stenosis on the same side (if I lean to the right and rotate to the right, I will produce stenosis on the right); thus, pathological nerve and venous compression and corresponding pain are generated. However, on the opposite side, traction is generated on the meningeal radicular sheaths. The pain, therefore, can have a bilateral distribution but with both nociceptive-compressive and meningeal characteristics. For example, there could be a radicular distribution on the side of the convexity and a diffuse lower back pain of a referred type on the side of the concavity. Add that the annulus of one or more vertebrae has been subject to abnormal torsions for years and can crack or protrude. In these cases, it may be challenging to recognise a flexor framework instead of an extensor one, both because of the structured deformity of the spine that does not give the patient many choices about the posture to adopt and because of the concomitance of a compressive (arthritic and venous) and traction (therefore meningeal) mechanism on the spinal roots. These often very difficult cases should be treated as lower back pain in both a

© The Author(s), under exclusive license to Springer Nature Switzerland AG 2025

L. Tesio, *Low Back Pain and Sciatica*, https://doi.org/10.1007/978-3-031-78534-4_10

flexor and extensor framework or with techniques that attempt to widen the stenotic areas and relax the meningeal traction.

A considerable physiotherapy experience is needed to treat these patients already affected by osteomuscular pathology. However, it's necessary not to abandon them to a diagnosis without hope based on a pure description of the deformity. Responding that 'the back cannot be straightened' is unacceptable. The pain arises because some drop has overflowed the vase. The treatment should not aim at the miracle of a new spine but allow a small step back that brings the situation to return asymptomatic. The drop must be removed, not the vase. An important detail is that deformity arises in adolescence, but the pain may never manifest or can manifest in adulthood. A patient-centered approach, understanding and addressing each patient's experiences and needs, is essential in these cases.

10.1.2　Pain in Malformations of Individual Vertebral Tracts

In these cases, analgesic-palliative or surgical-corrective interventions are usually necessary.

Like all median structures (from the nasal septum to the spinal cord to the bladder), the spine is subject to congenital alterations along its midline (dysraphisms). The column, moreover, can suffer from cranio-caudal alterations. There can be vertebrae that, in whole or in part, are not of the expected type but are typical of adjacent parts of the spine and are therefore defined as "transitional". There are dozens of possible segmental vertebral malformations, each quite rare and, in many cases, asymptomatic. A few rare but not exceptional conditions that could cause lower back pain will be mentioned below. These examples aim to alert the reader to the possibility that rare diagnoses underlie familiar symptom pictures and yet require unique treatments.

When it comes to diagnosing lower back pain, it's easy to fall into the trap of assuming that most cases can be explained by a few common diagnoses. However, this can lead to complacency and a lowering of the guard. The reality is that a minority of cases can hide a multitude of different diagnoses. The fact that these cases are rare should not be a reason to let our guard down. Given the high prevalence of lower back problems, it's likely that 'rare' cases can occur in any doctor's practice. This underscores the need for continuous learning and vigilance in practice, keeping the clinical audience motivated and alert in diagnosing and treating lower back pain.

10.1.3　Pain in Cases with "Transitional" Vertebrae

At the lumbar level, a sacralisation of the fifth lumbar vertebra or, conversely, a lumbarisation of the first sacral vertebra is common. If the "transition" is complete, the only problem is usually a difficulty in radiologically defining the level of a disc herniation: talking about a disc herniation at the L6/S2 level, for example, can generate confusion if the radiological report is not read carefully.

In my opinion, it's challenging for a lumbar spine that has been used to having only four vertebrae since birth to experience hypermobility when there's no fifth vertebra. Conversely, partial transitions can more easily generate pain. Here are three illustrative situations: the first is quite common, and the others are rare.

10.1.4 Pain in Transverse-iliac or Sacro-transverse Malformation

The pain arises from a mechanical conflict between a mega-apophysis of the fifth lumbar vertebra and the iliac wing or the sacrum. Sometimes, there is a fusion (and then we speak of hemi-sacralization of L5), but a pseudo-articular conflict is usually generated. The syndrome bears the eponym of the Italian physician Mario Bertolotti, who described it in 1917 [1]. The anatomical alteration, congenital but not necessarily symptomatic, is found in about 5% of the population.

The clinical picture can be that of lower back pain associated or not with sciatic reference. The mechanism that generates pain is varied and, in truth, not fully clarified. A unilateral or bilateral fusion generates hypermobility in the segment above (as in the case of surgical stabilisations). If the fusion is partial, the pseudo-joint produces typical arthritic symptoms. In this case, there should be an apparent tenderness to local palpation. In the case of fusion, a typical ASD—degeneration at above levels (see the case of stabilisations)- can benefit from techniques based on venous decongestion. The second case requires local treatment (infiltration with steroids and analgesics) of the pseudo-joint or surgical interventions (removal of the mega-apophysis or, on the contrary, lumbosacral fusion). An important detail: since the anomaly is congenital, this pain can occur at a young age.

10.1.5 Pain in Case of Abnormal Orientation of an Interapophyseal Joint

The orientation of the facet joints (*facet tropism*) is consistent with the movement of the adjacent vertebrae that contribute to the interapophyseal joint. It is not exceptional that, as a hint of a "transition", the facet joints on the two sides are oriented on different planes.

This anomaly generates continuous strains on the transitional interapophyseal joint. Due to the altered intervertebral dynamics, there seems to be an association between abnormal orientation, disc herniation and spondylolisthesis [2]. The pain is mainly local and does not fit into the CoVIn classification scheme, as it has an exclusively arthro-capsular origin. Conservative treatment, unfortunately, is only symptomatic and can extend to semi-invasive treatments such as infiltrations or sensory denervation of the facets (for example, with radio frequencies).

Normally, the lumbar facets have a different orientation for each vertebral pair and are distinct from the other spine sections. This orientation cannot be traced to the three "classic" orthogonal planes (sagittal, horizontal, frontal). As a rule, the articular surfaces are curved [3]. Simplifying, it can be said that the orientation of the lumbar facets favours flexion-extension and allows lateral flexion and rotation to a much lesser extent.

10.2   Pathogenesis in "Causeless" Pain

10.2.1 Theoretical Premise

In many cases, lower back pain does not seem justified, in whole or in part, by obvious biological causes or, according to an elegant Latinism, appears "sine materia" (non-material). In the dominant jargon, the pain is labelled as "non-organic" or, less brutally, as "functional". Often, this diagnosis implies a poorly disguised derogatory judgment ("the patient has nothing", "the pain is all in the patient's head").

The term "organic" represents one of the two poles of a consolidated dichotomy that sees the term "psychogenic" or "functional" at the other pole. Many different forms of chronic pain are labelled as sine materia: think of fibromyalgia, many headaches, and forms of dysmenorrhea. The unfortunate family of these conditions goes far beyond chronic pain of various kinds: think of chronic fatigue syndrome, a large part of psychiatric conditions and also disability, which in itself is a behaviour with very variable links to biological pathology [4]. The terminology that qualifies a condition of suffering as "sine materia" reflects philosophical positions that, like scientific ones, change over time: we go from the nineteenth-century term "hysteria" adopted by the great Jean-Martin Charcot, founding father of modern Neurology, who affirmed for hysteria the nature of a disease and not of simulation [5, 6], to the term "conversion" inspired by Freudian psychoanalysis, to arrive then at "somatisation" and finally, in recent years, to the term "neuro-functional disorder" that attempts a mediation at least linguistic between the two poles [7].

Another attempt at organic-psychic mediation is recognisable in the recent model of "nociplastic" pain, or a pain that tends to maintain itself even when the cause has disappeared, through synaptic maladaptation: a phenomenon, in truth, still to be demonstrated [8].

There is always an organic correlate of suffering (all perceptions and, in general, thought rest on nervous structures). Still, the difficulty arises in defining "cause" assigned to specific associations (for example, therapy-healing, disc herniation-pain, etc.): a rather complex philosophical problem. The problem simplifies if the goal is therapy. It must be accepted that in medicine, the "cause" is never unique, and above all, it often falls within a circular process, not a linear chain.

In the person, somatic pathology is associated with variable psychic modifications and psychic pathology is associated with variable somatic changes: it is not essential, for therapeutic purposes, to solve the egg-chicken dilemma. Think of a simplistic example like the obesity-depression association: do you become obese because you are depressed, or do you become depressed because you are obese? In Medicine (perhaps in all of Science), the link in this circular chain on which there are more possibilities of manipulation is called "cause". The general philosophical theme (the "ontology" of the cause) for a doctor can remain in the background. However, precisely identifying one or more target links is the task of scientific experimentation, which must be rigorous and conducted with specific methods concerning the therapeutic objective without prejudice. Otherwise, two equally serious errors can be made: aim only at psychological-relational diagnoses and therapies when the biological pathogenetic correlate (the "matter") is not transparent and therefore is filed as non-existent or, on the contrary, persist with attempts at diagnosis and "organic" therapies when psychological pathogenesis prevails [4, 9].

10.2.2 Pain Has Mainly Mechanical Causes; However, It Is Never Only Mechanical

My position is that, as a rule, chronic "benign" lower back pain, even when it appears "psychogenic", has mechanical causes (compressive and vascular) that interact with each other and are complicated by local inflammation. Therefore, according to the dichotomous terminology described above, it has an "organic" nature that is usually well recognisable. For example, the primarily "neuro-functional" patient rarely reports only lower back or sciatic pain while often reporting a more widespread "malaise" that is very inconsistent and variable in location, type, and intensity [9]. It is understood that the primarily neuro-functional patient who presents to the doctor for the treatment of back pain exists and should not be considered exceptional.

Like all unresolved chronic pains, however, lumbosciatic pain also generates psychological reactions that can be severe: in particular, anxiety about the associated disability (current or future), depression, and loss of self-esteem due to the countless previous, costly, and unsuccessful attempts at diagnosis and treatment. Indeed, these factors become causal links according to the circular model just exposed. Still, they are rarely a dominant cause, and it is exceptional that they are sufficient causes.

An "organic" trigger is often excluded due to interpretative deficiency. Even very modest instrumental results (protrusions or mild stenosis, for example, but "in the right place") can assume diagnostic significance if associated with motor behaviours (how to avoid or attenuate pain) and anamnestic data (onset and distribution of pain, response to certain types of drugs). All these signals are consistent with the hypothesis of an "organic" link that is easier to treat with conservative physical therapy than "psychic" links. The term "trigger" wants to underline that turning off even a modest but highly anxiety-provoking symptom can be more effective than an intense psychological intervention, primarily if the patient interprets "going to the psychiatrist" as giving up on a localised "organic" diagnosis. A diagnosis of the type "your pain is all psychological" can imply blame ("the problem is me, not my back"). It is common experience, for example, that patients with significant lumbar stenosis associated with modest symptoms are very frightened by the anxiety-provoking prognosis (usually unjustified) of "ending up in a wheelchair soon". No reassurance or anxiolytic therapy can be worth more than a therapy that - by attenuating claudication and pain - shows that the situation can be improved and is not doomed to become disastrous. However, psychiatric support on the "neuro-functional" links of the causal chain is often appropriate and should never be neglected: attacking two links is always better than attacking only one.

References

1. Quinlan JF, Duke D, Eustace S. Bertolotti's syndrome. A cause of back pain in young people. J Bone Joint Surg. 2006;88(9):1183–9.
2. Zheng Z, Wang Y, Wang T, Wu Y, Li Y, Khan R. A systematic review and meta-analysis of the facet joint orientation and its effect on the lumbar. J Healthc Eng. 2022;2022:2486745.
3. Bogduk N. Clinical and radiological anatomy of the lumbar spine. 5th ed. Edinburgh: Elsevier Churchill Livingstone; 2012.
4. Buzzoni M, Tesio L, Stuart MT. Holism and reductionism in the illness/Disease debate. In: Wuppuluri S, Stewart I, editors. From electrons to elephants and elections. Cham: Springer; 2022. p. 743–78.
5. Goetz CG. Charcot, hysteria, and simulated disorders. In: Hallett M, Stone J, Carson A, editors. Handbook of clinical neurology, vol. 139. New York: Elsevier; 2016. p. 11–23. Available from: http://www.sciencedirect.com/science/article/pii/B9780128017722000023.
6. Didi-Huberman G. The invention of hysteria. Charcot and the photographic iconography of the Salpetrière. Bologna: Dehoniano Publishing Center; 2020.
7. Demartini B, D'Agostino A, Gambini O. From conversion disorder (DSM-IV-TR) to functional neurological symptom disorder (DSM-5): when a label changes the perspective for the neurologist, the psychiatrist and the patient. J Neurol Sci. 2016;360:55–6.
8. Kumbhare D, Tesio L. A theoretical framework to improve the construct for chronic pain disorders using fibromyalgia as an example. Ther Adv Musculoskelet Dis. 2021;13:1–9.
9. Tesio L, Buzzoni M. The illness-disease dichotomy and the biological-clinical splitting of medicine. Med Humanit. 2021;47(4):507–12.

Part V

Macro-rationale of Non-surgical Therapy

Pain Therapies: Why They Are Not the First Choice

11

Pain therapy is a well-established discipline, practised mainly by doctors with an anesthesiological-resuscitation background. However, doctors from other backgrounds, such as oncological, rheumatological, neurological, and physiatric, also practice pain therapy. The term indicates an area of expertise that is relatively well-defined in the eyes of health professionals but not in those of patients.

Pain is, in most cases, a symptom of anatomically identifiable damage that primarily affects non-nervous tissues (nociceptive pain) or, directly, nervous tissues, central or peripheral (neuropathic pain) [1]. Unfortunately, the associated pathology is not always identifiable; even when it is, it is not always eradicable (think of some neoplastic pains). Pain, therefore, remains the only attackable link in the causal chain: from symptom, it becomes a disease.

The 'pain therapist' employs a comprehensive approach, utilising traditional pharmacological means, instrumental physical therapies, and semi-invasive therapies such as joint infiltrations, epidural endoscopic infiltrations or lysis, denervations with radio frequencies, and the implantation of spinal electro-stimulators or infusion pumps. My impression is that there is an excessive recourse to this fundamental discipline by patients with benign chronic lumbar pain. As a rule, these are the many patients who see "pain therapy" as a last resort because they have not found a solution to their problem with the most varied conservative or surgical therapies.

In cases where an "organic" cause is recognisable (for example, disc herniation or interapophyseal arthrosis), the most varied therapies have been unsatisfactory. In other cases, the diagnosis has remained nebulous (or simply that of psychogenic disorder), and the patient seeks refuge in those who appear expert in dealing with the symptom as such. The questions to ask are whether the patient has reached the last resort in pursuing a cause of pain and consequent therapy and whether delegating the problem to 'pain therapy' does not represent evidence of a diagnostic-therapeutic inability that has emerged in previous approaches.

© The Author(s), under exclusive license to Springer Nature Switzerland AG 2025

L. Tesio, *Low Back Pain and Sciatica*, https://doi.org/10.1007/978-3-031-78534-4_11

Reference

1. Raja SN, Carr DB, Cohen M, Finnerup NB, Flor H, Gibson S, et al. The revised International Association for the Study of Pain definition of pain: concepts, challenges, and compromises. Pain. 2020;161:1976–82.

Exercise Therapies and Manual, Instrumental Physical or Pharmacological Therapies

12.1 Treatment Rationale for the Flexion Pattern

With the metaphorical term "clinical picture", we want to highlight the importance of "how the patient appears". According to the convention adopted in this text, the flexion pattern is, therefore, that of the patient who finds relief in trunk flexion (or in general in "de-lordotization" of the lumbar spine) or who does not feel a worsening in flexion while feeling pain, or who worsens, in extension. As mentioned above, this patient typically has pain with the maintenance of prolonged postures that favour venous stasis and even more typically when getting up from bed in the morning and in general in postural changes as long as after periods of immobility (supine-sitting, sitting-standing). Therefore, the mechanism that generates pain is narrowing the lumbar canal through the vicious circle between compression (nervous and venous), epidural venous dilation and further compression.

12.2 How to Decompress Without Surgery

12.2.1 The Flexion Exercise

Exercise cannot anatomically lengthen the spine. Still, it can flatten its curves: the "flexor" or "self-stretching" exercises widen the vertebral canal and are the cornerstone of a conservative approach. The historic Williams exercises, already mentioned, are suitable for home self-administration after brief teaching by the physiotherapist. However, the exercise techniques used mainly require the active intervention of the physiotherapist, who performs passive mobilisations or against resistance. Significant professional competence and also considerable ingenuity in personalising the treatment are needed.

© The Author(s), under exclusive license to Springer Nature Switzerland AG 2025

L. Tesio, *Low Back Pain and Sciatica*,
https://doi.org/10.1007/978-3-031-78534-4_12

The mechanism of action is not only that of widening the canal: something that would make the benefit very transient. The exercise causes stretching[1] of muscles often shortened because of an overall reduced mobility muscles (of relevance here, the extensor muscles, both superficial and deep) and joint capsules and ligaments, all now adapted to chronic shortening. Likely, there is also an adaptation of the neuromuscular spindles; therefore, latent hypertonia tends to recede. The "contracted" and painful muscles that characterise many clinical cases probably reveal a contraction that would like to be defensive, limiting the movements of the spine, but then becomes itself a source of pain. The contracted muscle eventually becomes ischemic and, therefore, painful.

This explains why treatments must be repeated (indicatively, a "cycle" involves at least 8–10 sessions in 2–4 weeks). The aim is to make a less lordotic lumbar spine position easier and more frequent. This is nothing new compared to established manual mobilisation techniques (applied, for example, to limb joints after post-traumatic immobilisation) that involve muscular and ligamentous stretching—even if this is not the stated objective.

12.3 How to Decongest Without Surgery

12.3.1 Still, the Flexion Exercises

The flexion exercise has already been said to facilitate venous decongestion by widening the lumbar canal. In reality, any active exercise of the paravertebral musculature can act the same way as long as – like the flexion exercise – it does not involve the narrowing of the vertebral canal. The same applies, in general, to an aerobic type of exercise (for example, cycling or running). However, immersion in thermoneutral water gives an even more specific decongestant effect, as seen in the next paragraphs.

12.3.2 Extensor Exercises: No Thanks

Are extensor exercises preferable? It should be noted that a model of exercise based on the assumption that in most cases of benign chronic low back pain, the extension of the spine pushes the pulpy nucleus forward and attenuates the pain is very influential. I am referring to the model published by New Zealand physiotherapist Ron McKenzie in 1981 [1]. The model is disc-centric and has its pivot in a defined framework of *derangement*. Extension exercises, both passive and active, would achieve an anterior displacement of the disc and the posterior detension of the

---

[1] It should be remembered that stretching lengthens the muscle belly, not the tendon. The tissue to be lengthened is the connective one, which wraps in parallel the contractile matter (fasciae, peri- and endo-mysium). The contractile matter will also lengthen, inserting new sarcomeres in series so that the greater joint excursion does not translate into excessive shortening of the individual sarcomeres, causing, in this way, loss of strength.

annulus, which would thus have a way (if overstretched or fissured) to repair. Ideally, the manoeuvres should cause pain that, however, should disappear when the forced extension ceases.

In his manual, McKenzie cites several contradictory articles based on anatomical imaging that do not appear to contemporary eyes to prove the hypothesised disc dynamics. Today, we know that the hypothesis is wrong and that in a disc in the initial degenerative phase, the extension of the spine involves posterior disc protrusion (see the dedicated paragraphs). McKenzie also distinguished a syndrome of *dysfunction*, caused by the compression of soft tissues and attenuated by the removal of the load, and a *postural* syndrome, caused by a retraction of soft tissues due to prolonged improper positions, generating pain if the spine is brought to whole stroke. Moreover, this important author admitted that there could be (for him rare) derangement syndromes in which it was appropriate to flex the lumbar spine to push the disc fully to the stop.

More generally, the method emphasises a *treatment principle*. In the case of derangement, this consists of respecting the direction in which the treatment manages to reduce the pain or manages to "centralise" it towards the lumbar area when there is sciatica or, in the case of dysfunction, force the movement in the direction in which the pain increases. In this second case, the aim is to produce greater extensibility of the tissues. This partially flexible strategy, therefore, aims, through cycles of repeated sessions, to repair damaged tissues (like a fissured annulus) or to bring overstretched tissues (for example, due to an annulus overstretched by a disc protrusion) back to normal stiffness, or to bring retracted tissues (joint capsules, ligaments and interspinous muscles) towards greater extensibility.

The "McKenzie method" is very structured; it has extended to dorsalgia and cervicalgia and has generated official "McKenzie Institutes" in many countries. The fact that it is based on an anatomical model that is no longer consistent with anatomical knowledge and somewhat limited (the suffering disc would protrude anteriorly in extension, which does not happen; neither venous stasis epidural nor meningeal pain is considered) does not in itself exclude that the empirical solution is effective: think of the history of active lumbar traction to which we will refer shortly. The method appears in total contrast with the CoVIn model but, more importantly, the few studies with a control group that have addressed the effectiveness of the technique have not shown superiority over a treatment with flexor exercises [2] nor the ability to reduce the recourse to herniectomy [3]. A recent Cochrane review defines the method simply as ineffective [4].

It should be emphasised, however, how research in the sector is complicated not only for specific problems in behavioural research, including physiatric [5], but also, in the specific case, for the lack of a shared model of classification of patients whose pain is often framed under the standard label of "non-specific" [6]. The CoVIn model has at least the advantage of dividing cases into "flexors" and "extensors" according to a rationale that does not prioritise anatomical alterations that can be documented with images or neurological signs. As we have seen, imaging and neurological signs are somewhat unpredictably correlated with pain and the effectiveness of therapies.

12.3.3 Exercise in Water

For centuries, the "thermal bath" has been used for various diseases, including in rehabilitative medicine (for a recent study, see Maccarone et al., 2023 [7]). Here, we will not consider the therapeutic properties of the chemical characteristics of the waters nor the effect of various temperatures but the physical effects of immersion in thermoneutral water, or 33.5–34 °C, and with a density close to that of water of lakes and rivers, tap water, or of swimming pool (i.e., slightly above 1 g ml^1). At this temperature, there is no physiological reaction to the temperature itself. Other physiological effects, however, are not lacking. First, there is the buoyancy force (or Archimedes' principle), which is proportional to the volume of the immersed mass and the density of the water. Therefore, one can relieve body weight, which can already be helpful for rehabilitative purposes (for example, in traumatic aftermath, rheumatoid arthritis, and muscle weakness of various natures). This "lightening" can also explain, at least in part, the notorious muscle relaxation that thermo-neutral immersion entails, despite the presence of gravity. Another interesting phenomenon is the viscous resistance opposed by water to body movements, which is proportional to their speed. The patient can graduate the muscular power required by an exercise simply by modulating its speed.

But let's now come to the most interesting mechanism, the "venous squeezing". Immersion causes a compression proportional to the depth and density of the immersion liquid. The muscles of the lower limbs and trunk (particularly the abdomen) are compressed. Therefore, an "elastic stocking" effect is obtained in a few seconds, squeezing a considerable amount of additional blood towards the right atrium [8]. In a man about 1.80 m tall, the cardiac volume during upright standing can increase from about 560 ml to 800 ml when the water reaches the armpits, as inferred from Fig. 12.1 [9].

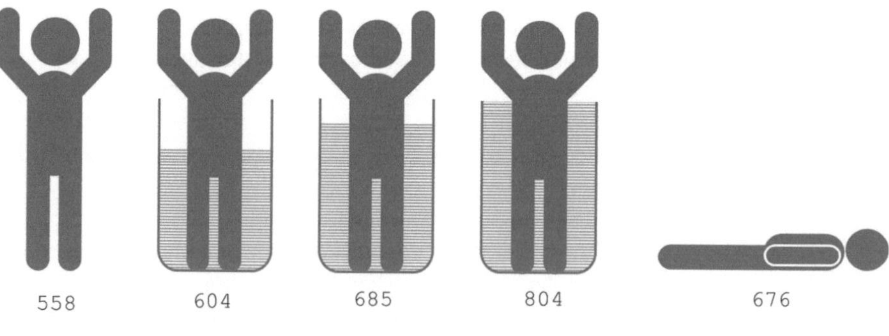

Fig. 12.1 Variations in cardiac volume in immersion. Cardiac volume is in the standing position (image on the left end), in the supine position (picture on the right end), and according to various degrees of static immersion (the three central figures). Six healthy subjects. Average values: age 23 years; height 1.83 m; weight 73 kg (modified by Risch et al. [9], with permission)

This is a physiological reaction to hypervolemia that does not exist: there is only a redistribution of the blood already present in the venous system. The distended (not in failure) heart increases its contractile power (Starling's law); consequently, the heart rate decreases (even by 20%), systolic pressure increases, diastolic pressure decreases, and diuresis increases. But there's more: atrial distension increases the secretion of atrial natriuretic hormone and, through vagal afferents, inhibits the hypothalamic secretion of antidiuretic hormone. In practice, a physiological diabetes insipidus is generated [10]. Suppose the immersion is prolonged for at least 20–30 min. In that case, there is also a "squeezing" of interstitial fluid towards the venous circulation that offers partial compensation for the hypovolemia induced by the increase in diuresis. This influx reduces plasma density and viscosity (the hematocrit also drops by 4–5 percentage points) [11, 12]. These phenomena are well-known in human physiology, particularly cardiovascular and respiratory pathophysiology. Some have proposed a tub suitable for immersion treatments [13].

The possible indications for a short immersion treatment range from lymphedema to cases of heart failure, ascites from liver cirrhosis, high blood pressure, and (unsurprisingly) varicose veins and oedema of the lower limbs in pregnancy [14–16]. The effectiveness of immersion increases if flexor exercises are combined with buoyancy. In hospitals and rehabilitation centres, however, immersion remains very rare. Immersion therapy ("balneotherapy") is applied mainly in spas.

12.3.4 Associating Other Manual or Instrumental Therapies

Therefore, the "flexor" exercises[2] and immersion remain the dominant traditional ingredients of the therapeutic program inspired by the CoVIn model. However, for the above reasons, this program can include other manual techniques (massages, manipulations) and instrumental physical therapies (thermotherapies, electrotherapies) aimed at the paravertebral muscles. However, the therapeutic logic must remain that of facilitating decompression, not just aiming at analgesia.

---

[2]The study of immersion is also an essential topic in neurophysiology and aerospace medicine because, in some respects, immersion simulates the absence of gravity (or, more appropriately, microgravity: some gravitational field in the universe is always found). Here, we can only mention the fact that, notoriously, the absence of gravity, eliminating hydrostatic pressure, leads to a more homogeneous redistribution of body fluids (from which, for example, the typical "puffy" appearance of astronauts returning to Earth after stays in microgravity). It is known that the volume of the intervertebral discs also increases due to excessive hydration, a phenomenon that can significantly facilitate, upon return, the formation of painful disc hernias. The phenomenon has been reproduced with "dry immersion" experiments for 3 days in beds with water mattresses at 33 °C. Fortunately, disc swelling does not occur with short periods of immersion, such as those required by therapies, which are less than 45 min.

12.4   The Whole Model in One Method: Active Lumbar Traction (or Autotraction)

Active Lumbar Traction (ALT) is the name I assigned in 1992 to the original technique of "Autotraction" (Autotraktion in the original Swedish, Autotraction in English). I will dedicate a considerable space to this technique for two reasons. The first reason is historical: my first reflections on the pathogenesis of lumbosciatic pain arose following the direct finding of the effectiveness of this technique in the face of its disarming simplicity and, above all, in the face of a paradoxical increase in disc pressure. The second reason, instead, is its significant support of the CoVIn model: central support in this text because at the moment only the CoVIn model offers a rational explanation for the effectiveness of ALT.

12.4.1 The Active Lumbar Traction Bench

The technique uses a specially designed physiotherapy bench divided transversely into two equal sections. Each section can be tilted up or down and rotated to the right or left through an electric servo mechanism controlled by the physiotherapist. The bench has transverse bars placed above the surface at the end of each section. The patient is anchored to the caudal section through a pelvic belt and a chain (hence the name - as will be seen, clinically misleading - of "traction") (Fig. 12.2). The patient can "pull" himself towards the cranial end of the bench by clinging to the cranial bars above his head. Pushing against the caudal bars or anchoring himself to them with the back of his feet, the patient can favour the traction exerted with the upper limbs or oppose it, or even, by extending the knees, add a selective flexion of the pelvis and the lumbar spine. The push or unilateral traction with a lower limb induces lateral flexion or torsion of the pelvis and, therefore, of the lumbar spine. The prone position is rarely used as it is often poorly tolerated.

12.4.2 How Treatment Is Performed

Depending on local regulations, a medical prescription may be necessary. The patient lies supine on the table. The physiotherapist moves the table sections and identifies the least and the most painful positions. Starting from the least painful positions, the physiotherapist asks the patient to exert maximal "self-traction" efforts for about 5–6 s and then gradually relax in a few seconds. This is followed by a pause of about 20–40 s (or more if the patient requests it). The cycle is repeated. The entire session lasts a maximum of 30 min. During the effort, the patient is asked to inhale (which is not always spontaneous), but exhalation can also be accepted. However, a Valsalva manoeuvre (i.e., "holding" the breath) should be avoided. The self-traction manoeuvre must not generate either the onset or increase of pain.

During the effort or the breaks, the physiotherapist modifies the spine's position, moving it towards the initially more painful positions. These manoeuvres must

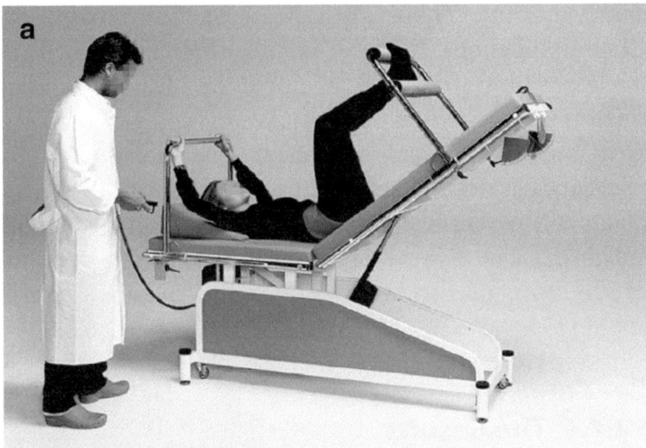

Fig. 12.2 The table for active lumbar traction. On the left is a typical initial treatment position, with the lumbar spine flexed or with reduced lordosis (**a**). On the right (**b**): the typical final position of a treatment session is with the lumbar spine extended. The basic concept of the session is to start with the least painful positions and to lead the patient through "self-traction" manoeuvres to free themselves from pain in the painful positions [17]

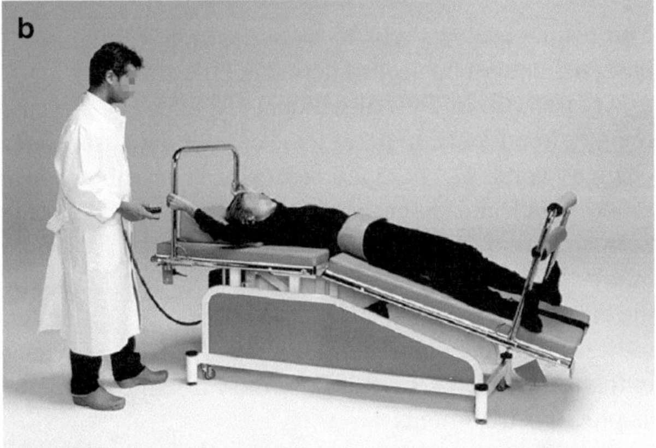

"free" the positions gradually conquered from pain. The treatment can also be effective in cases where there is no clear distinction between painful and non-painful positions. The logic is to start from flexion and then move towards extension. Of course, you can also work on lateral flexions (patient on one side) and the twists of the spine through flex-extensions and axial rotations of the bench caudal section or by associating asymmetric pushes and pulls with the lower limbs.

Typically, a session is performed every 2–3 days. The pain should decrease after the third session (curiously, sometimes 5–7 days later). In this case, I proceed with another 3–6 sessions to try to "free" the entire lumbar joint range. No prevention or "maintenance" procedure is needed if the treatment succeeds.

12.4.3 Indications and Contraindications

The indications are extensive. They range from cases with evident disc herniations to cases of lumbar stenosis and to cases of patients who have had unsatisfactory surgery, even those with surgical stabilisations (in which cases, spine mobilisation is minimised). There must be a medical diagnosis of "benign" lumbar pain. Contraindications, however not absolute, include risks associated with efforts with the upper limbs (cervical or shoulder pathology) and increased abdominal pressure (therefore also central venous). We can mention the presence of abdominal hernias or prolapses, ventriculoperitoneal derivations, painful varices or thrombophlebitis. Pregnancy is not in itself an absolute contraindication, nor is the presence of transplants (for example, a kidney transplanted into the iliac fossa). In these cases, body anchoring can also be obtained only through dorsiflexion of the feet against the caudal bars of the table. A specific manual describes the technique in more detail [17].

12.4.4 The Results

The results are very positive and lasting. This appears to be a pathophysiological paradox, as will be seen. There can be a reduction in pain of at least 70% (however it is measured) in 75% of patients [18–23], even in cases of chronic pain refractory to other treatments, including the case of pain associated with noticeable anatomical changes (multiple hernias, stenosis). The same applies to post-surgical epidural scars, which are essentially a post-surgical fibrotic process that incarcerates the lumbar roots [24]. My experience with over 5000 patients over 35 years confirms that even the total disappearance of pain is widespread and, another paradox, that the effectiveness is long-lasting, on the order of many months [21] or years (in anectodical cases, even decades). Recurrences probably occur in less than 10% of cases in the following 5–10 years, and their treatment has the same probability of success as previous treatments.

The literature with imaging reports favourable remodelling of the disc profile [25, 26] as well as instrumental evidence of a neurophysiological effect (reappearance of osteo-tendinous reflexes, of normal skin temperature and of somatosensory evoked potentials in the limbs that presented sciatica) [27]. However, another paradox is that the prognosis does not seem to be linked to the "objective" severity of the clinical pictures [18, 26]. The results of Tesio et al. and the previous ones of Lind, Natchev and other Swedish authors [21, 26] seem to overlap. Tesio et al. report the significant effectiveness of lumbosciatica in pregnancy [19, 28], a frequent condition 34 that has never found a clear pathophysiological framework.

12.4.5 How the Technique of ALT/Autotraction Was Born (And Why it Did Not Spread)

The technique was first proposed in 1974 by the Swedish doctor Gertrud Lind [25], who died prematurely. The original table was manually operated. Later, a Bulgarian surgeon who was naturalised Swedish and a disciple of Lind, Emil Natchev, perfected the bench by adding a system of electrically operated hydraulic pistons. He formalised the method, which remained very complex, in a dedicated manual and spread the technique through intensive courses and seminars [29].

In 1984, I attended one of Natchev's courses in Stockholm, imported a bench to Milan, and greatly simplified the technique [23, 30] and the bench design.[3] I dubbed the method Active Lumbar Traction for the reasons that will be clarified below. A physiotherapist can learn the method in 2 days. Thanks to a collaboration with neurosurgeons of the National Neurological Institute Carlo Besta [19] also in Milan, there was immediate evidence of effectiveness, significantly superior, for example, to that of treatments with conventional passive traction [18, 21–23]. The latter can have only transient effectiveness, not superior to a placebo [31].

12.4.6 Too Many Paradoxes?

The mechanism of action of the ALT appeared immediately somewhat contradictory. Lind believed that her Autotraktion acted by distancing the vertebral bodies as it was thought that the traditional passive pelvic tractions acted, with the addition of a classic principle of Manual Medicine, namely the selective positioning of the spine in a painless position [32]. In addition, Lind argued that the technique could "bring back" significantly the disc protrusions [25], as she had demonstrated with myelography in some cases. The method worked, but the interpretive model was partly wrong.

Around the 1960s of the last century, the famous Swedish orthopaedic surgeon Alf Nachemson developed a technique for measuring in vivo lumbar disc pressure [33] and since then proposed the dogma ("disc-centric" like all Medicine after the already mentioned works of Mixter and Barr) according to which positions and activities of the spine that increase disc pressure should be proscribed as risk factors, if not direct causes, of lumbosciatic pain. In the 1980s, a group of important Swedish authors (including Nachemson) found themselves faced with the paradox of having to admit the effectiveness of "active" traction [22] and having demonstrated that the same manoeuvre increased disc pressure [34]. This should not surprise: in "pulling" with the upper limbs, the patient intensively contracts the paravertebral and abdominal muscles. Nachemson arbitrarily resolved the paradox in favour of a complete rejection of Autotraction.

The theoretical model, therefore, resisted and prevailed over experimental evidence (a frequent and well-known error in Medicine and Science in general) [35, 36]. Add to this that the evidence of direct action on the morphology of disc protrusions was somewhat controversial (we are in an era of onset for CT, and preceding MRI). Moreover, it was already evident that the method's effectiveness was very little influenced by the radiological and clinical severity of the case, another apparent paradox. Finally, neither Lind nor Natchev were academic authorities that could compete with Nachemson's prestige.

---

[3] The ALT table is produced in Italy by Chinesport SpA, Udine - www.chinesport.it (accessed on January 4th, 2025).

The recall of the technique's name to "traction" certainly did not help, as the scientific community does not particularly appreciate passive traction. I changed the technique's name to "active lumbar traction" - ALT to mitigate this unfavourable factor. ALT is essentially a form of active exercise, not passive traction. In support of this, there have been two isolated reports of the effectiveness of "self-traction" exercises that do not use the dedicated bench [20, 37].

The Swedish school's adverse judgment, consistent with the dominant disccentric view of benign lumbosciatic pain, contributed decisively to the method's limited diffusion. The absence of academic mentors did the rest. The treatment with "Autotraktion" remained popular only in Scandinavian countries but did not arouse further experimental interest, except for the recovery I carried out in Italy in 1985/1995. Since 1995, scientific production on the subject has been stagnant. In Italy, the technique remains marginally known and little practised.

12.4.7 The Mechanism of Action: No Longer Paradoxical

The effectiveness of active lumbar traction no longer appears paradoxical within the CoVIn model, and indeed, it supports it.

The paravertebral contraction is associated - an important detail - with a selective lumbar spine arrangement at the beginning of the treatment: this is to widen its section. The position likely favours venous outflow from areas where it generates compression or ischemia. Furthermore, remodelling of the disc-nerve interface cannot be excluded, as it is sufficient to decompress algogenic terminations without causing noticeable alterations to the disc profile. Therefore, ALT probably acts mainly on epidural venous congestion and significantly on the hernia profile. For this reason, it could act with a combined mechanism very similar to exercise in water despite the diversity of procedures.

Gradually "freeing" the entire lumbar excursion demonstrates to the physiotherapist that the manoeuvres have been effective enough to make even potentially compressive positions painless. However, the question remains: why would these positions be useful for treatment since they do not widen or narrow the vertebral canal? It is possible (but empirical experience makes it unlikely) that manoeuvres in a flexed position are sufficient. Two hypotheses can be made for now. The first hypothesis assumes that the treatment adds venous outflow to the slackening of the dural sac, of which a modest irritation can never be excluded. The second hypothesis assumes that the positions in extension, once made painless, favour further venous"squeezing" in the conjugation foramina and the roots' initial extraforaminal path.

12.4.8 Venous Pathogenesis: It's Time for Imaging

It must be admitted that there is still a lack of targeted experimentation to demonstrate the association between clinical improvement and changes at the epidural venous level. Standard imaging techniques with CT or MRI are not aimed at the epidural venous plexus, which is never considered the object of a specific diagnostic question. It seems that the plexus can be well studied in vivo with MRI, with or without contrast medium, as demonstrated by the eloquent three-dimensional images provided by a radiological study on patients before and after surgery on lumbar stenosis [38]. The same type of study would, therefore, not only be possible but also desirable to highlight the effect of conservative treatments on Batson's venous plexus.

12.4.9 Let's Not Forget Drugs

12.4.9.1 Drugs "For Pain"

Nothing prevents also aiming at common analgesic or anti-inflammatory treatments. However, it should be borne in mind that in the case of benign chronic pain, the pain itself should be considered primarily a symptom and much less a disease. The doctor can, therefore, associate classic NSAIDs or paracetamol, for example. Personally, in "flexor" cases, I only exceptionally prescribe steroids (usually reserved for "acute" extensor cases) or opioids. I only exceptionally prescribe muscle relaxants or drugs for neuropathic pain (such as gabapentin, pregabalin, and tricyclics) as the pain is almost always of a nociceptive type. There may be an indication for these latter drugs in cases of sciatica or cruralgia with precise radicular distribution (radiating pain), but always remember that the best therapeutic (and not just symptomatic) goal is decompression.

The prescription may include psychotropic drugs in cases where "neurofunctional" symptoms predominate, but this is a much broader topic of the treatment of chronic pain, which has already been mentioned.

12.4.10 "Vascular" Drugs: From Pain to its Causes. Why Not?

Given venous insufficiency's leading role in the CoVIn model, a brief reflection on a possible therapeutic role of drugs now well established for the treatment of venous insufficiency and phlebitis is appropriate: antithrombotic heparins (for example, sulodexide) and flavonoids (for example, oxerutin). The former also have a fibrinolytic effect and, therefore, seem indicated not only in venous and capillary endothelial protection but also in treating epidural fibrosis.

I am not aware of published trials on the efficacy of this type of drug in chronic low back pain. Still, according to the CoVIn model, there seems to be already a rationale for their use—a rationale that would be interesting to reinforce with specific experimentation. "Venous" drugs could complement conservative motor, physical, pharmacological, and even post-surgical therapies. In some cases of mild lower back pain, they could even be proposed as the first-choice attempt.

12.5   Treatment Rationale for the Extensor Picture

12.5.1 Rest and Dexamethasone

In this text, much more emphasis is given to the flexor picture than the extensor one. The reason has already been expressed: the "extensor" patient is usually not chronic and is much rarer. The pain - typically of acute and recent onset - is very intense (the classic "witch's blow") but tends to regress spontaneously in a few days. Some cases with neurological signs may also require emergency surgery, but this is another story. In the dedicated paragraph, an attempt was made to demonstrate how this pain is of meningeal origin. Lumbar extension narrows the vertebral canal and causes posterior protrusion of the disc (especially the annulus) and excessive overlap and pressure between the facet joints. On the other hand, extension relaxes the dural sac, attenuating the dominant meningeal pain.

In my opinion, these cases, which are not chronic, should be treated with rest and—whenever clinically possible—with steroids. It is not advisable to choose any steroid but dexamethasone, which has the maximum anti-oedema effect. Dexamethasone is well known to neurologists and neurosurgeons, who apply it at high doses in many conditions of cerebral oedema.

I prescribe 4 or 8 mg/day of dexamethasone through intramuscular injection, even in a single administration, for 3–4 days. I usually prescribe gastroprotection but without then proceeding to décalage in the following days. Suppose you want to follow a chronobiological rule. In that case, it is better to administer the steroid in the morning between 7 and 9 and then in the evening around 5 in the case of twice-daily injection. The pain should recede quickly (in 6–12 h) and could give way to a typical flexor picture. Otherwise, the case must be reviewed from the beginning. The persistence of any strength deficit with radicular distribution requires a surgical opinion.

References

1. McKenzie R, May S. The lumbar spine mechanical diagnosis & therapy. 2nd ed. Wellington: Spinal Publications; 2003.
2. Elnaggar IM, Nordin M, Sheikhzadeh A, Parnianpour M, Kahanovitz N, Kahanovitz N. Effects of spinal flexion and extension exercises on low-back pain and spinal mobility in chronic mechanical back pain patients. Spine. 1991;16(8):967–72.
3. Kilpikoski S, Häkkinen AH, Repo JP, Kyrölä K, Multanen J, Kankaanpää M, et al. The McKenzie method versus guideline-based advice in the treatment of sciatica: 24-month outcomes of a randomised clinical trial. Clin Rehabil. 2024;38(1):72–84.
4. Almeida MO, Narciso Garcia A, Menezes Costa LC, van Tulder MW, Lin CWC, Machado LA. The McKenzie method for (sub)acute non-specific low back pain. Cochrane Database Syst Rev. 2023;4(4):CD009711.
5. Tesio L. 6.3B. Scientific background of physical and rehabilitation medicine: specificity of a clinical science. J Int Soc Phys Rehabil Med. 2019;2(Suppl 1):S113–21.
6. Balagué F, Mannion AF, Pellisé F, Cedraschi C. Non-specific low back pain epidemiology and natural history. Lancet. 2012;379:482–91.

7. Maccarone MC, Magro G, Albertin C, Barbetta G, Barone S, Castaldelli C, et al. Short-time effects of spa rehabilitation on pain, mood and quality of life among patients with degenerative or post-surgery musculoskeletal disorders. Int J Biometeorol. 2023;67(1):29–36.

8. Risch WD, Koubenec HJ, Gauer OH, Lange S. Time course of cardiac distension with rapid immersion in a thermo-neutral bath. Pflfigers Arch. 1978;374:119–20.

9. Risch WD, Koubenec HJ, Ulrich B, Lange S, Gauer OH. The effect of graded immersion on heart volume central venous pressure pulmonary blood distribution and heart rate in man. Eur J Physiol. 1978;374:115–8.

10. Epstein M. Renal effects of head-out water immersion in humans: a 15-year update. Physiol Rev. 1992;72(3):563–621.

11. Grossman E, Goldstein DS, Hoffman A, Wacks IR, Epstein M. Effects of water immersion on sympathoadrenal and dopa-dopamine systems in humans. Am J Physiol. 1992;262(6 Pt 2):R993–9.

12. Yamazaki F, Endo Y, Torii R, Sagawa S, Shiraki K. Continuous monitoring of change in hemo-dilution during water immersion in humans: effect of water temperature. Aviat Space Environ Med. 2000;71(6):632–9.

13. Epstein M, Norsk P, Loutzenhiser R, Sonke P. Detailed characterization of a tank used for head-out water immersion in humans. J Appl Physiol. 1987;63:869–71.

14. Pechter U, Maaroos J, Mesikepp S, Veraksits A, Ots M. Regular low-intensity aquatic exercise improves cardio-respiratory functional capacity and reduces proteinuria in chronic renal failure patients. Nephrol Dial Transplant. 2003;18(3):624–5.

15. Katz VL, Rozas L, Ryder R, Cefalo RC. Effect of daily immersion on the edema of pregnancy. Am J Perinatol. 1992;9(4):225–7.

16. Smyth RMD, Aflaifel N, Bamigboye AA. Interventions for varicose veins and leg oedema in pregnancy. Cochrane Database Syst Rev. 2015;2015(10):CD001066.

17. Tesio L, Merlo A, Raschi A. Active lumbar traction. Physiopathological and clinical review. Guidelines for treatment. Ric Riabil. 1996;1:1–28.

18. Tesio L, Merlo A. Autotraction versus passive traction: an open controlled study in lumbar disc herniation. Arch Phys Med Rehabil. 1993;74:871–6.

19. Tesio L, Luccarelli G, Fornari M. Natchev auto-traction for lumbagosciatica: effectiveness in lumbar disc herniation. Arch Phys Med Rehabil. 1989;70:831–4.

20. Ljunggren AE, Weber H, Larsen S. Autotraction versus manual traction in patients with pro-lapsed lumbar intervertebral disc. Scand J Rehabil Med. 1984;16:117–24.

21. Gillstrom P, Ehrnberg A. Long-term results of autotraction in the treatment of lumbago and sciatica. Arch Orthop Trauma Surg. 1985;104:294–8.

22. Larsson U, Choler U, Lidstrom A, Nachemson ALF, Nilsson B, Roslund JAN. Auto-traction for treatment of lumbagosciatica. Acta Orthop Scand. 1980;51(5):791–8.

23. Tesio L. Autotraction treatment for low-back pain syndromes. Crit Rev Phys Rehabil Med. 1995;7(1):1–9.

24. Benoist M, Ficat C, Baraf P, Cauchoix J. Postoperative lumbar epiduro-arachnoiditis: diagnostic and therapeutic aspects. Spine. 1980;5(5):432–6.

25. Lind G. Auto-traction treatment of low-back pain and sciatica. Linkoping: University of Linkoping; 1974.

26. Gillström P, Ericson K, Hindmarsh T. Autotraction in lumbar disc herniation - A myelographic study before and after treatment. Arch Orthop Trauma Surg. 1985;104(4):207–10.

27. Knutsson E, Skoglund CR, Natchev E. Changes in voluntary muscle strength, somatosensory transmission and skin temperature concomitant with pain relief during autotraction in patients with lumbar and sacral root lesions. Pain. 1988;33(2):173–9.

28. Tesio L, Raschi A, Meroni M. Autotraction treatment for low-back pain in pregnancy: a pilot study. Clin Rehabil. 1994;8:314–9.

29. Natchev E. A manual on auto-traction treatment for low-back pain. Stockholm: Tryckeribolaget i Sundvall AB; 1984.

30. Tesio L, Merlo A, Raschi A. Active lumbar traction. Scientific review. Manual. Treatment guidelines. Ricerca in Riabilitazione. 1996;1:27–45.

31. Wegner I, Widyahening IS, van Tulder MW, Blomberg SEI, de Vet HCW, Brønfort G, et al. Traction for low-back pain with or without sciatica. Cochrane Database Syst Rev. 2013;2013(8):CD003010.
32. Maigne R. Pains of vertebral origin. Understand, diagnose and treat. New York: Elsevier; 2009.
33. Nachemson A, Morris JM. In vivo measurement of intradiscal pressure: discometry, a method for the determination of pressure in the lower lumbar discs. J Bone Joint Surg. 1964;46-A(5):1077–91.
34. Andersson GBJ, Schultz AB, Nachemson AL. Intervertebral disc pressures during traction. Scand J Rehabil Med. 1983;15(Suppl. 9):88–91.
35. Barber B. Resistance by scientists to scientific discovery. Science. 1961;134(3479):596–602.
36. Kuhn TS. The structure of scientific revolutions (Original edition 1962). Turin: Einaudi; 2009.
37. Bonaiuti D, Gatti R, Raschi A, Cantarelli L, Sirtori V. Manual autotraction: preliminary study on the effectiveness of a new device for back pain treatment. Eura Medicophys. 2004;40:75–81.
38. Kamogawa J, Kato O, Morizane T. Three-dimensional visualization of internal vertebral venous plexuses relative to dural sac and spinal nerve root of spinal canal stenosis using MRI. Jpn J Radiol. 2018;36(5):351–60.

Reflections on Conservative Therapy

13

A macro-rational can now be proposed for prescribing conservative therapies. We must refer to Fig. 8.1, which schematises the CoVin model. This model, as we have seen, is quite simple. I will not discuss pharmacological therapy further, which can be a valuable complement to mechanical interventions. Nor will I only return to surgical treatments, which are within the competence of physiatry and physiotherapy for some of their outcomes.

13.1 Diagnosis: From Descriptive to Pathophysiological

The purpose of this text, as anticipated at the beginning, is not to provide a review of the anatomy and pathology of the spine nor to provide operational suggestions for treating this or that patient. The text wants to give an update on pathophysiological concepts related to a widespread syndrome that is still defined in a generic and purely descriptive way. Sooner or later, this condition will no longer be described as "non-specific" and perhaps not as "back pain". We will have to find other more pathophysiological and specific definitions. I venture some examples, including imaginative acronyms: "mechanical lumbar pain from extradural compression" (MLP-EDC?), "mechanical lumbar pain from meningeal irritation" (MLP-MI?), "lumbar pain from chronic epidural phlebitis" (LP-CEP?). We will see…

13.2 Therapeutic Deductions: Three Model-compatible Techniques

I have provided three macro-indications for a non-invasive treatment, yet not only symptomatic: Williams-type flexor exercises (and derivatives), water exercise and active lumbar traction. Having applied them for many years, hopefully, I have

© The Author(s), under exclusive license to Springer Nature Switzerland AG 2025

L. Tesio, *Low Back Pain and Sciatica*,
https://doi.org/10.1007/978-3-031-78534-4_13

grasped their effectiveness and a common and solid rationale despite their differences.

At this stage of knowledge on the subject, I would say that their effectiveness, evident empirically, supports the CoVin model. Conversely, if the model is established, new techniques can be inspired by it.

It should be remembered that all these techniques aim to create space within the vertebral canal. Venous decongestion is an essential component of this program. What mechanism supports the stability of the results? In any physiotherapy on the musculoskeletal system, the stability of the results is based on better mobility that can maintain the greater muscle-ligament extensibility achieved. In the case of lumbar pain, however, stability is also based on venous decongestion, which, as already mentioned, is the requirement to interrupt a thrombophlebitic-fibrotic process.

13.3   From the CoVin Model to Clinical Decision: The Step Is Short

The CoVin model, with its bifurcation (flexor frame vs. extensor frame), provides a much simpler classification tree compared to the numerous classifications in the literature for benign chronic lumbosciatalgia [1]. This bifurcation serves as a guide for therapeutic decision-making. Subsequently, the focus shifts to determining the most effective treatment or combination of treatments. These decisions, however, are still awaiting robust experimentation.

For example, we do not know if, in the case of a flexor frame, it is advisable to apply active lumbar traction (which I consider the first-choice treatment) alone or together with simple vertical immersion or associated with exercises, or together with "dry" flexor exercises, or with pharmacological or electro-analgesic treatments. In the case of association, we do not know if applying the different therapies in the same period or succession is advisable. However, these issues are not particularly urgent, given the simplicity and non-invasiveness of the three types of treatment proposed.

My proposal does not aim to exclude technical improvements to these methods. The fields of physiatry, physiotherapy, and healthcare in general are often burdened with obsolete therapeutic models, many of which are identified with historical eponyms. While these models have been crystallised for decades, they should not be considered unchangeable. Instead, they should be open to evolution and improvement, guided by new research and clinical experience.

Therefore, the purpose of this book is primarily to stimulate critical reflection on an interpretive theoretical model and, no less importantly, to stimulate new ideas and research projects. My bibliography is extensive and covers a broad period, but I know it remains deficient. I encourage the readers to critically engage with the material and contribute to the ongoing discourse in this field.

Therefore, I have added a brief "Appendix" related to tricky clinical cases. This is not because the topics I have included are marginal but because I think the appendix will be the section that will most probably need to undergo updates and expansions in the event of new editions: I might as well start.

Therefore, readers can conclude the book here unless they are interested in clinical refinement that can aid them in their jobs. I welcome any criticism or feedback, as it will contribute to the ongoing development and refinement of the ideas presented in this book.

Reference

1. Stynes S, Konstantinou K, Dunn KM. Classification of patients with low back-related leg pain: a systematic review. In: BMC musculoskeletal disorders, vol. 17. London: BioMed Central Ltd; 2016.

Appendix - Some Treacherous Causes of Low Back Pain

When the Numbers Don't Add Up

The 'chronic benign' lower back pain to which the text is dedicated has been reduced to two primary and antagonistic paradigms, the 'flexor' and 'extensor' framework. As already anticipated, it is evident that they do not cover the entire range of intermediate and mixed frameworks, let alone cover the peculiarities of many benign clinical situations. These, although essentially benign, like those based on already mentioned malformations, do not fall under the CoVIn model. The case histories are infinite but unfortunately, the published case reports always struggle to become systematic knowledge: this was seen in the case of the many reports of 'varicose' epidural, which remained orphaned of a taxonomic recognition in the context of a more general 'phlebopathy of the epidural plexus'. I will, therefore, only point out a few clinical situations that are not supported by causes attributable to the spine, but that might seem so. This is to stimulate the maintenance of vigilance on the part of the clinician even when his cases of low back pain accumulate, and risk seems all alike.

Lower Back Pain in Adolescents or Children

Osteoid Osteoma

Disc herniations are rare, but not exceptional, before age 20. However, during the period of bone growth, one must not forget the osteoid osteoma, which prefers growth cartilages. If the osteoma originates from a vertebral pedicle and projects into a conjugation foramen, it can generate antalgic scoliosis to dilate the obstructed foramen. The solution is surgical. Take home message: never skimp on magnetic resonance imaging of the spine if a child or teenager is afflicted with lower back pain.

The treacherous osteoma can also appear below the peroneal head. The irritation of the adjacent external popliteal sciatic nerve generates a causalgia (like carpal tunnel syndrome) that can extend between the thigh and leg in a territory approximately attributable to the L5 radicular level. One must consider this

© The Editor(s) (if applicable) and The Author(s), under exclusive license to
Springer Nature Switzerland AG 2025
L. Tesio, *Low Back Pain and Sciatica*, https://doi.org/10.1007/978-3-031-78534-4

diagnosis if a lumbosacral MRI is negative. For the diagnosis, a knee x-ray is enough, which may seem absurd in a case of "sciatica". In this case, too, the solution is surgical.

Spondylolysis-spondylolisthesis

A spondylolysis can be seen at 6–7 years old and become symptomatic several years later, but it can also remain asymptomatic. A significant spondylolisthesis (on bilateral lysis) is rare at this age. If it causes pain, the spondylolysis does so in extreme excursions of the spine. Probably, the lysis/listhesis started with trauma, but the history is difficult to recover. Think about it anyway. An MRI should be enough for the diagnosis, but it is not said. If the suspicion persists, in addition to the usual anteroposterior, lateral and oblique X-rays, a lumbar CT scan may be necessary. The radiologist should be alerted to the clinical suspicion because the orientation required for the "CT cuts" can be specific. The appropriate solution, conservative or, in extreme cases, surgical, should aim at stabilising the hypermobile segments (a topic beyond this book's scope).

Suffering of the Piriformis and the Internal Obturator Muscle

The small, deep pelvitrochanteric muscles are not familiar to doctors. Let's mention two: piriformis and internal obturator [1]. The piriformis syndrome is probably over-diagnosed and is characterised by a type of sciatic pain as well as pain on deep gluteal compression, if not also during the simple sitting position (there are then manoeuvres to sensitise the compression, but this is another story [2]). However, one never thinks about the suffering of the internal obturator muscle, which has a particular anatomical course. Its tendon runs on the ischial branch posteriorly, like on a pulley. Therefore, it can easily remain compressed in the case of gluteal trauma (the classic "fall on the buttocks"), even if mild. The pathogenesis then resembles that of suffering from the rotator cuff of the shoulder (subfascial hematoma and then muscle fibrosis). Still, the symptoms are very elusive: they range from deep groin pain to gluteal pain to crural pain, all accentuated by unpredictable hip movements. We must think about it: the main examination is an MRI of the pelvis that a specific question in the request must accompany. In the pelvis, there is everything, and the radiologist's attention must be directed. The solution can be entrusted to manual or infiltrative medicine.

"Primitive" Gluteal Pain

The buttocks are the site of radiated or more frequently referred pain, attributable to pain originating at the vertebral level L4 or L5. A pain only in the buttock can fall within the CoVIn model. However, care must be taken when, after a fall "on the buttocks," a sudden gluteal pain is observed, even very modest, associated with a sudden strength deficit: it could be a case of entrapment of the superior gluteal nerve between the piriformis and the great ischial notch. This results in immediate paralysis of the abductors (gluteus medius and tensor of the fascia lata) and is usually reversible in a few weeks. From a neurophysiological point of view, a conduction block prevails, caused by severe temporary demyelination with modest associated axonal damage (a picture that, however, cannot be demonstrated electromyographically before 2–3 weeks) [3]. The solution is to wait.

In rare cases, gluteal pain, with gradual onset, can be of vascular origin (buttock claudication), although usually, it is expected that vascular claudication produces distal symptoms [4]. The syndrome should be recognised because the pain only increases with walking (when the buttocks claim blood supply), especially uphill, and only beyond a certain walking distance. The high intensity of the pain and its restricted location should differentiate this syndrome from a spinal claudication from a narrow lumbar canal. The solution is biological competence (the cause must be sought in an obstruction in the aortic or iliac artery territory).

Pain at the Iliac Crest

The iliac crest and the adjacent upper gluteal area can be sites of very localised pain, which typically increases with local palpation. For several decades, a syndrome of suffering of the superior cluneal nerves caused by entrapment between the thoracolumbar fascia and the iliac crest has been described. The superior and medial cluneal nerves are sensory branches of the posterior branch of the spinal nerves that originate from the lumbar roots and T12. Although much more limited, the area of pain (and possibly of allodynia or hypoesthesia) overlaps with that of typical "sciatic" pain. The diagnosis remains clinical and is indirectly based on the exclusion of radicular suffering and the effectiveness of possible infiltrations with steroids, possibly targeted with ultrasound guidance. This condition is rare (unlike radicular suffering L4 or L5). Still, it is also true that it is a diagnosis that is little thought of (for a recent review, see the work of Anderson et al. [5]).

Sacroiliac Pain

The literature takes for granted that from 15% to 30% of benign chronic low back pain originates from a dysfunction of the sacroiliac joint (true joint and/or sacroiliac ligament), even in non-traumatic cases. By dysfunction, we mean substantially uni- or bilateral hypermobility with instability. In my opinion, the existence of this condition is at least doubtful, not less than vertebral instability. Even admitting a causal role for this "dysfunction", I consider its prevalence highly overestimated. One should remember that the sacroiliac area is the site of referred and radiated pain from the L4, L5 and S1 segments. Also, at the moment, the diagnosis of sacroiliac pain does not seem to be based on instrumental findings (including MRI), which usually do not show any alteration. The diagnosis is based on the response to injections in the suspected joint: either an anaesthetic that attenuates the pain or a contrast medium that increases it. Alternatively or in combination, the diagnostic criteria require the positivity of at least three of the six most well-known provocative manual manoeuvres (among the many publications on the subject, I only mention a few [6–10]). The diagnosis, therefore, consists of a precarious self-confirmatory procedure: causing local pain does not prove that spontaneous pain originates from the same site; the effect of an anaesthetic can be widespread; controlled studies with placebo procedures or control are lacking. However, manual therapy of the sacroiliac joint is very practised in physiotherapy and in the context of osteopathy and chiropractic.

Chronic sacroiliac pain, in my opinion, should initially be considered a very persistent aftermath of traumatic injury; for example, compound sacral fractures (often not very evident in X-ray and MRI but evident in CT) are frequent after falls in osteoporotic people. If pain appears during pregnancy, perhaps (I doubt it) one can think of a physiological ligamentous laxity. Suppose there is no history of trauma (and pregnancy is not ongoing). In that case, it is reasonable to think of rheumatic diseases (from psoriatic arthritis to ankylosing spondylitis to Paget's disease and others). Septic or neoplastic localisations should not be forgotten. Pregnancy aside, in all these cases, there is instrumental evidence consistent with an underlying pathology much less "benign" than the hypothetical "dysfunction": evidence that must be sought without settling (and often without need) for provocative manoeuvres, whether they are manual or infiltrative.

Hyperacute Pain with Different Antalgic Positions

There may be the case (sporadic) of a patient who is "blocked" instantly by very intense lumbar pain, even without having made particular efforts: a case that does not fall into the "extensor" framework (and therefore in the CoVIn model) referred to in the previous chapters nor a framework of meningeal pain. For example, the "blocked" patient may prefer a position of the trunk flexed and rotated to the right instead of extended and retroflexed to the left. The MRI may not show any alteration (for example, an expelled hernia) that explains the clinical condition. These may be among the rare cases for which a manipulation manoeuvre (of exclusive medical competence) is indicated.

What could be the pathogenesis? At the upper and lower poles of the facets, the joint capsule presents a fibro adipose pad (a "meniscoid") covered by synovia that facilitates sliding. In addition, the meniscoid protects the joint surface that remains uncovered during the relative movement of the facets. In the movements of mutual distancing of the facets, a cartilage fragment can be "torn" from the meniscoid, and - when the overlap is restored - the fragment gets stuck in the joint [11]. From this event arises a very acute pain associated with strong muscle contraction that immobilises the segment in the position - quite variable and unpredictable - that minimises intra-articular compression.

The manipulative manoeuvre (the so-called thrust mentioned in the note in Chap. 3) perhaps acts by reflexively inhibiting muscle contraction and expelling the incarcerated tissue. The thrust can be associated with a "cracking-popping" sound. The sound does not indicate bone collision but joint decompression followed by the exit and bursting of nitrogen bubbles dissolved in the synovial fluid. The cracking sound has a powerful placebo effect ("they put my back in place"), but in reality, it is not essential: for example, it is less intense or absent if the joint has moved previously, preventing a high diffusion of nitrogen in the synovial fluid.

In any case, the crack phenomenon confirms the hypothesis that manipulation also acts through joint decompression, and in this case, the only joints involved are the inter-apophyseal ones. Before proceeding with the thrust, the doctor must verify the presence of at least one direction in which the trunk can move freely and force the movement in that direction [12]. The benefit, if any, must be immediate and then persistent.

References

1. Martinoli C, Miguel-Perez M, Padua L, Gandolfo N, Zicca A, Tagliafico A. Imaging of neuropathies about the hip. Eur J Radiol. 2013;82(1):17–26.
2. Michel F, Decavel P, Toussirot E, Tatu L, Aleton E, Monnier G, et al. Piriformis muscle syndrome: diagnostic criteria and treatment of a monocentric series of 250 patients. Ann Phys Rehabil Med. 2013;56(5):371–83.
3. Tesio L, Bassi L, Galardi G. Transient palsy of hip abductors after a fall on the buttocks. Arch Orthop Trauma Surg. 1990;109(3):164–5.
4. Tago M, Hirata R, Oda Y, Katsuki NE. Buttock claudication: what induces pain only in the left buttock on every movement? BMJ Case Rep. 2019;12(6):e231271.
5. Anderson D, Szarvas D, Koontz C, Hebert J, Li N, Hasoon J, Viswanath O, Kaye AD, Urits I. Comprehensive Review of Cluneal Neuralgia as a Cause of Lower Back Pain. Orthopedic Reviews. 2022;14(3):1–10.
6. Buchanan P, Vodapally S, Lee DW, Hagedorn JM, Bovinet C, Strand N, et al. Successful diagnosis of sacroiliac joint dysfunction. J Pain Res. 2021;14:3135–43.
7. Liu Y, Suvithayasiri S, Kim JS. Comparative efficacy of clinical interventions for sacroiliac joint pain: systematic review and network meta-analysis with preliminary design of treatment algorithm. Neurospine. 2023;20(3):997–1010.
8. Schwarzer, Anthony C, April CN, Bogduk N. The sacroiliac joint in chronic low back pain. Spine. 1995;20(1):31–7.
9. Szadek KM, van der Wurff P, van Tulder MW, Zuurmond WW, Perez RSGM. Diagnostic validity of criteria for sacroiliac joint pain: a systematic review. J Pain. 2009;10:354–68.
10. Dreyfuss P, Dreyer S, Griffin J, Hoffman J, Walsh N. Positive sacroiliac screening tests in asymptomatic adults. Spine. 1994;19(10):1138–43.
11. Bogduk N. Clinical and radiological anatomy of the lumbar spine. 5th ed. Edinburgh: Elsevier Churchill Livingstone; 2012.
12. Maigne R. Pains of vertebral origin. Understand, diagnose and treat. New York: Elsevier; 2009.

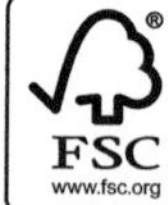

MIX
Papier aus verantwortungsvollen Quellen
Paper from responsible sources
FSC® C105338

If you have any concerns about our products,
you can contact us on
ProductSafety@springernature.com

In case Publisher is established outside the EU,
the EU authorized representative is:
Springer Nature Customer Service Center GmbH
Europaplatz 3, 69115 Heidelberg, Germany

Printed by Libri Plureos GmbH
in Hamburg, Germany